ALSO BY HEALTH FOR LIFE

ISBN 0-944831-36-2

Library of Congress Catalog Card Number: 95-62164

HEALTH FOR LIFE

8033 Sunset Blvd., Suite 483–Los Angeles, CA 90046–(800) 874-5339

1 2 3 4 5 6 7 8 9

THE BODY BALL BOOK

THE BODY BALL BOOK

BY JAN PRINZMETAL & BRIAN SHIERS

A
SYNERGISTIC
WORKOUT
FOR THE
LOWER BODY

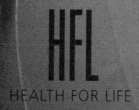

HEALTH FOR LIFE

CREDITS AND ACKNOWLEDGMENTS

EDITORS

Robert Miller & Jerry Robinson

BOOK DESIGN

Jerry Graves Design

PHOTOGRAPHY

Michael Neveux

WARNING

Contents

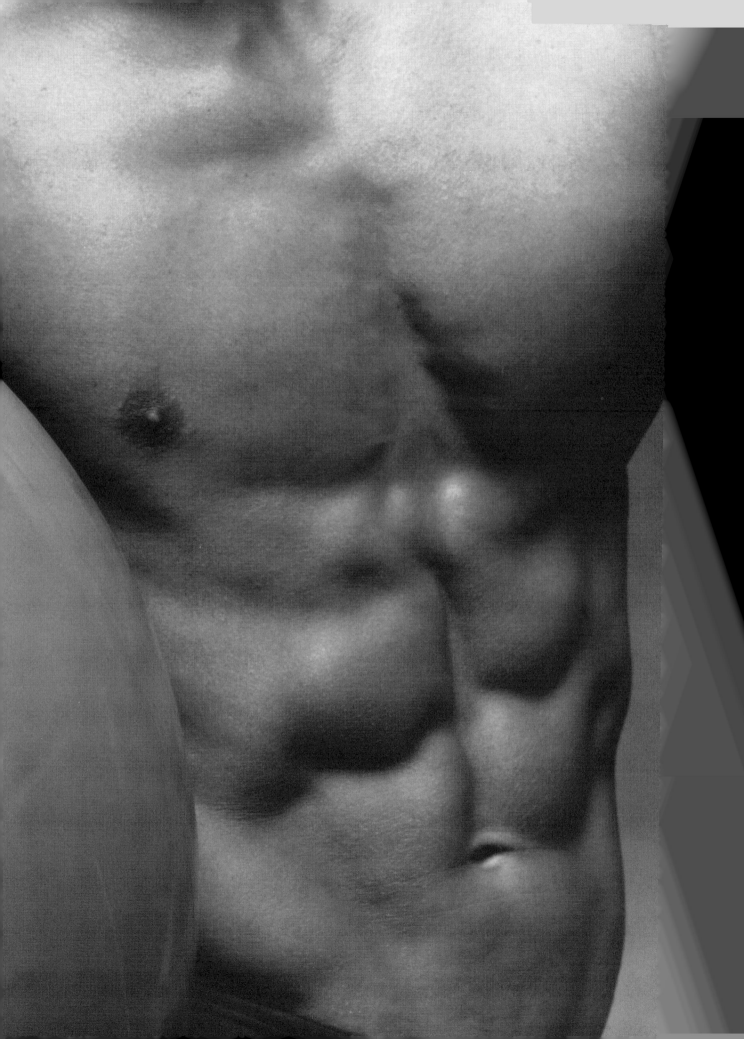

The Body Ball Book

C O N T E N T S

XIV

XV

Introduction

Introducing the Body Ball — a new workout device that can help anyone develop a tighter, leaner, stronger lower body!

The Body Ball (also known as *Physio-, Soma-, Swiss-,* or *Gymnastik Ball*) has been an essential tool for physical conditioning since 1965, when Swiss physical therapists began using it to help their patients develop balance and maintain reflex response. Since then, a growing number of physical therapists in the U.S. have begun to incorporate the Ball into their rehab routines. Now the Body Ball is available as a conditioning tool for home use.

How can the Ball help you? Body Ball training is an inexpensive, safe, and effective way to dramatically tighten and tone your thighs, hips, buttocks, and abdominals. Plus, it's fun!

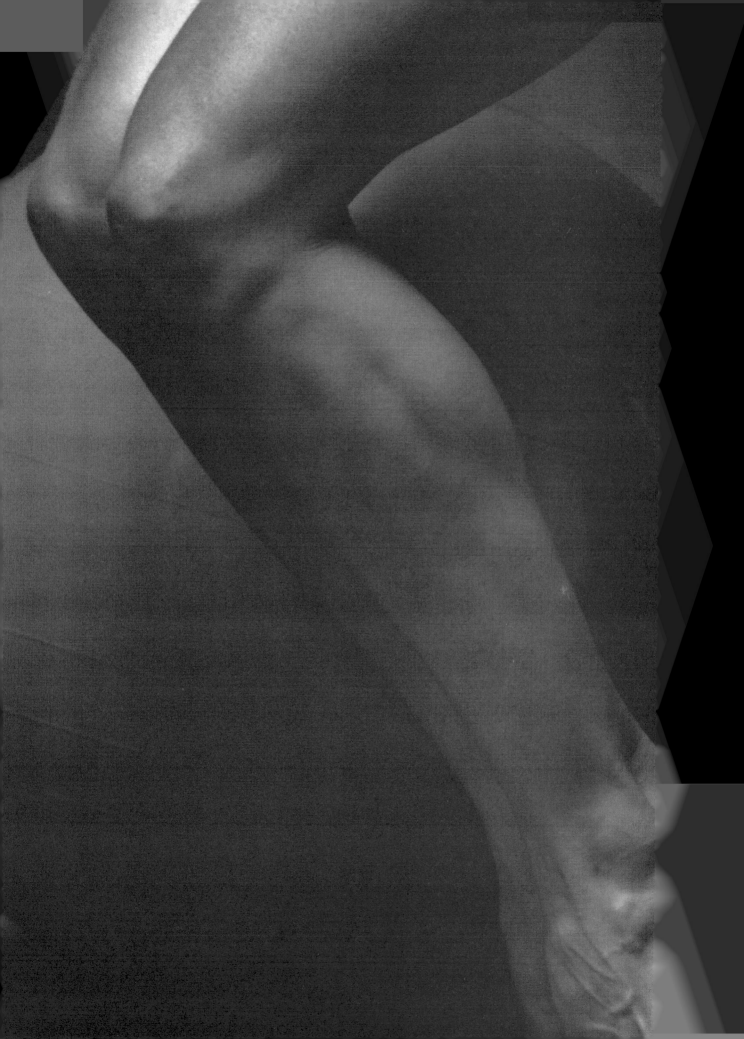

The power of the Ball lies in its versatility. By lying, bouncing, or rocking on the ball in a variety of postures, you can effectively stretch, warm up, tone, and strengthen all the lower body muscles. Many of the exercises shown here would otherwise require expensive, cumbersome equipment, and quite a few can only be performed with the Ball.

The Body Ball Book employs the same synergistic training concepts that underlie all *Health For Life* programs. Each exercise has been carefully adjusted for maximum efficiency and biomechanical soundness. Many were developed by HFL and are presented here for the first time. Most important, these exercises have been arranged into a synergistic routine — adjusted for optimum sequence, timing, and numbers of sets and reps. The result is the first complete, scientifically designed program for working out on the Body Ball: a program guaranteed to condition your lower body and abdominals in as little as 15 minutes per session!

What's Coming Up

Chapter 1: *Preliminaries* — Basic concepts to help you get the most out of the *Body Ball Routine*

Chapter 2: *The Exercises* — Detailed performance guidelines for the exercises that serve as building blocks for the routine

Chapter 3: *The Body Ball Routine* — Five levels ranging from beginning to advanced, plus a *How Much, How Often* section that lays out your optimum schedule

Preliminaries

This chapter will cover some simple, but powerful, exercise

principles. Taking a few minutes to understand them will go far

toward ensuring you get the fastest results possible with the

HFL Body Ball Routine.

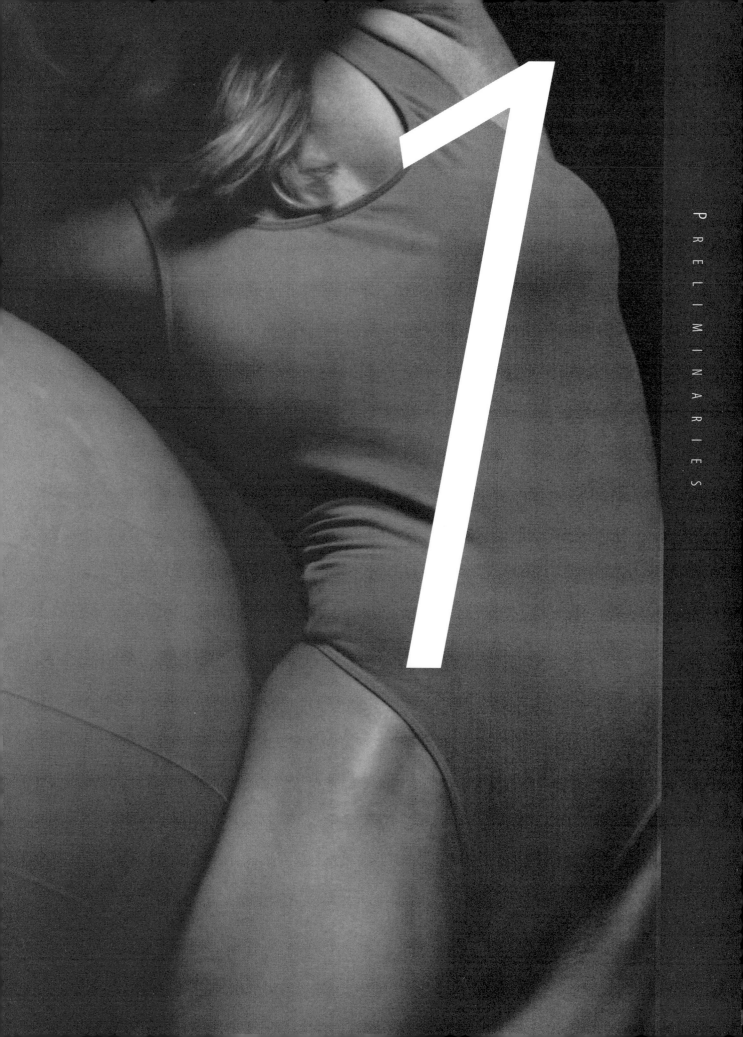

1

To start off, we'll take a look at four major workout concepts — **Resistance and Reps**, **Exercise Form**, **Sequence**, and **Pace**. These are the physical and physiological nuts and bolts of any good exercise program. In particular, we'll explain how each of these elements can be optimized for maximum results.

Resistance and Reps

As a rule, the exercises done as "floor work" in an aerobics class usually require 20 to 30 repetitions or more. This can be quite tedious. What's more, it's not necessary! If your goal is to tone and strengthen muscles, the most efficient way to do it is by using high-resistance exercises that require fewer reps to overload the muscle.

HFL's Body Ball program uses your bodyweight to create resistance — the Ball itself is essential in helping to put your body in positions you couldn't otherwise achieve. The exercises are designed to create an overload within a minimum number of reps. When exercises become too easy, instead of simply adding more reps, you move to new exercises, or to a more difficult arrangement of exercises. Helping you achieve this progression is the purpose of the *Routine* chapter.

Exercise Form

Working with good form saves time and effort. But what makes good form "good"? The key to proper form is *body position* — specifically, a position that precisely matches the *motion of an exercise* to the *action of the muscle* being targeted.

Think of a car jack. Since the weight of a car pushes straight down, the jack must be positioned to push straight up or it can't do its job. In the same way, there is only one body alignment for a given exercise that pits the force created by your muscles directly against the resistance. Doing an exercise with good form means doing it without deviating from this ideal position.

The Body Ball Book does the technical work for you: Each exercise in this program is designed to match motion to muscle action as closely as possible. Beyond that, mastering the subtleties of performance is up to you. By understanding the relationships of the muscles to their movements, you can make appropriate adjustments to your performance — changing the the placement of the feet, angle of the body, and so on — so that the small details all contribute to an optimum workout.

You'll find muscle diagrams and explanations later in this chapter to help you.

Before you begin to work out, read the instructions for each exercise in *Chapter 3* carefully and take time to develop a "feel" for the muscle being targeted. Each rep should be done slowly and deliberately through the greatest possible range of motion. If you feel any sharp or unusual pain, stop immediately.

Sequence

Does the order in which you do a group of exercises really make a difference? *Absolutely*. In fact, this factor alone can turn a mediocre routine into a exceptional one!

To understand the role exercise sequence plays in *The Body Ball Book's* routine, you need to know the difference between **isolation** exercises and **functional strength** exercises and how they interact to fatigue a target muscle.

ISOLATION AND FUNCTIONAL STRENGTH EXERCISE

Isolation exercises and functional strength exercises represent opposite ends of a spectrum. Isolation exercises strive to limit your efforts to a single target muscle; functional strength exercises involve many muscles. There are benefits to both. Isolating a muscle is the fastest, most direct way to work it and gives you great control over the overall development of your physique. Functional strength exercises are beneficial from a health standpoint, as they condition you for actions in everyday life. Functional strength exercises also elevate your metabolic rate more than isolation exercises, resulting in more calories burned *between* workouts.

In fact, though, there is no such thing as a true isolation exercise — an exercise that works one muscle and one muscle only. Other muscles *always* participate to some degree, either by helping the main muscle perform the motion or by stabilizing the body while the motion occurs.

Nevertheless, the fewer assisting muscles, or **synergists**, involved in an exercise (and the less they assist), the more that exercise *acts* as an isolation exercise. Likewise, the more assisting muscles involved (and the more they contribute), the more a movement acts as a functional strength exercise.

How does the distinction between isolation and functional strength exercise affect your workout?

MUSCLE INTERACTION AND EXERCISE ORDER

Most body parts can be conditioned using either functional strength or isolation exercises. Often, though, people will do exercises for a certain muscle group without any regard for which category they fall into — i.e., whether they involve other muscles and if so, how this involvement affects the target muscle. Random arrangements of exercises like this are a poor substitute for a cohesive program.

The fact is, exercise sequence matters a great deal! You can significantly boost —or significantly diminish — the value of your workout just by rearranging the exercises.

For example, suppose you're training the gluteal muscles, and you're planning to do both Wall Squats (page 24) and Glute Bridges (page 29). Which should you do first? You should do Glute Bridges first — here's why:

Starting with Wall Squats (a functional strength exercise with many muscles involved), gets your glutes tired — but only slightly, because so many other muscles assist. Following up with Glute Bridges increases the fatigue, but still only moderately, because the glutes aren't that tired before you begin the second exercise.

On the other hand.... *Starting* with Glute Bridges (a virtual isolation exercise for the glutes and hamstrings), tires the glutes *significantly* right off the bat. Then, when you follow up with Wall Squats, you put them well over the top — because all those assisting muscles keep you going beyond the point at which the glutes would give out if they were acting on their own. This is called **pre-exhausting** the glutes. Result: You get a much more intense workout in the same amount of time!

This approach to sequencing is one of the key principles behind our routines. By taking into consideration the various muscles' roles as prime mover or synergist in each exercise, we are able to vary the difficulty level of the routines — without having to add unnecessary extra reps — just by carefully rearranging the sequence.

The power of this technique will become obvious once you try it!*

Pace

Many potentially good exercise programs are compromised because they don't reflect the importance of workout **pace**.

Simply put, resting less is generally better — because, while you do need to recuperate between efforts (especially if you're a beginner), you need far less rest than you might think. In fact, for continued progress, you must push the fatigue of each target muscle past a certain level and keep it there until you finish working that muscle.

Generally, for greatest results, rest only 15 to 30 seconds between sets and 30 to 45 seconds between exercises. You'll find more specific recommendations in the *Routine* chapter.

Some HFL programs recommend that functional strength exercises come before isolation exercises rather than after, as described here. The theory in this book derives from special considerations that apply when creating a bodyweight program, as opposed to a machine- or free-weight program.

When setting out to condition muscles, it's beneficial to learn a little about where they are and how they function. This knowledge will help you fine-tune your form so you can work most effectively.

As you read the following descriptions, try to locate each muscle group in your own body and perform the associated movements to get a feel for their their actions.

The Gluteal Group (Buttocks)

The **gluteals**, or *glutes*, consist of the **gluteus maximus**, **gluteus medius** and **gluteus minimus**. With the help of several smaller muscles, the glutes act to create motion at the hip joint. The gluteus maximus, largest of the group, runs from the crest of the pelvis, spreading to the side and down, forming the general curve of the buttocks. Its primary function is to straighten (or extend) the hip. It also serves to rotate the hip outward.

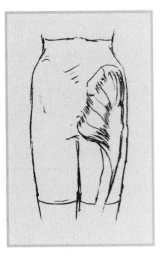
Gluteus Maximus

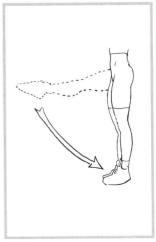
Extends the hip

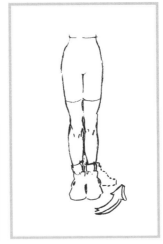
Rotates the hip outward

PRELIMINARIES

The gluteus medius, the next largest of the gluteal group, is located just below and to the rear of your hip bone. The medius is responsible for rotating your leg inward (internally rotating the hip) and, with help from the gluteus minimus and other muscles, lifting your leg to the side (abducting the hip).

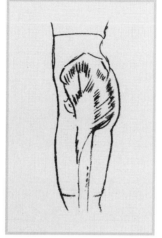

Gluteus Medius

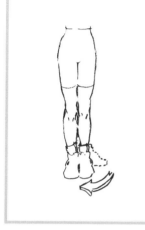

Rotates the hip inward

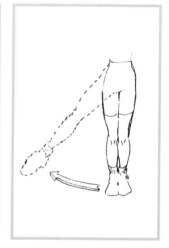

Lifts the leg out to the side

The Quadriceps Group

The front of your thigh comprises four separate muscles called the **quadriceps**, or *quads*, which all cooperate to straighten (extend) the knee. One of these, the **rectus femoris**, also helps to raise your thigh (flex your hip), as in the action of walking.

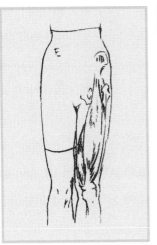

Quadriceps

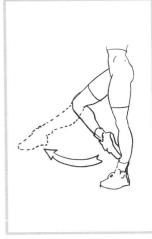

Straighten the knee

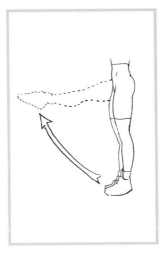

The rectus femoris also raises your thigh

The Adductor Group

The **adductors** run along your inner thigh and pull your leg in toward your midline (adduct the hip).

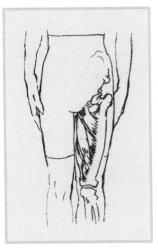

Adductors

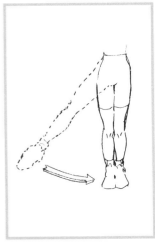

Pull the leg inward

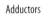

P R E L I M I N A R I E S

The Hamstrings Group

The **hamstrings** run along the backs of your thighs and work in opposition to the quadriceps by bending (or flexing) the knee. In addition, some members of the hamstring group also assist in drawing the hip backward (extending the hip).

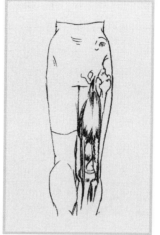

Hamstrings

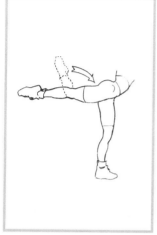

Bend the knee

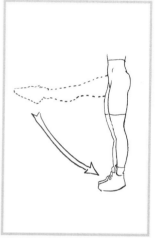

Extend the hip

The Calf Muscles

The calves are primarily made up of two muscles of the lower leg: the **gastrocnemius**, the most visible of the two, and the **soleus**, which runs just beneath it. Both are responsible for pointing your toes as you rise onto the balls of your feet (plantar flexion).

(See illustration on next page)

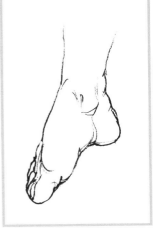

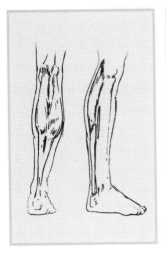

Gastrocnemius / Soleus

Point the toe

The Spinal Erectors (Lower Back)

The **spinal erectors** are the two parallel bands of muscle that run along either side of your lower spine. They straighten your back (extend the spine). To ensure the health of your back, these muscles must be kept strong and flexible.

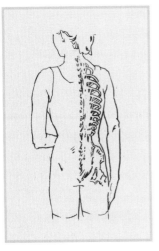

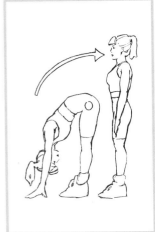

Spinal Erectors

Straighten the spine

CHAPTER 1

The Abdominal Group

The complimentary muscles to the spinal erectors — equally important for the stability and health of the lower back — are the **abdominals**, or *abs*. The largest member of this group is the **rectus abdominis**, which runs vertically from rib cage to pubic bone. Its primary function (in a lying position) is to bend the trunk up to 30 degrees (flex the spine). Other muscles in the abdominal group include the **internal** and **external obliques**, which wrap around the sides of the trunk and act to twist the torso (rotate the spine). They also assist the rectus abdominis in flexing the spine. When overdeveloped or covered with fat, the obliques are often referred to as *love handles*.*

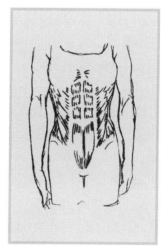 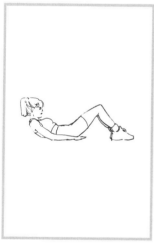 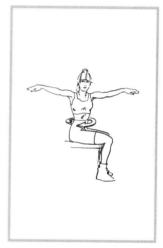

Abdominals   Round the spine   Rotate the torso

❖ ❖ ❖

A little time invested in studying and understanding the relation of these muscles to their motions will pay off as you begin doing the exercises. This knowledge will also help you if you decide to experiment with new exercises of your own.

There is a fourth muscle in the abdominal group — the transversus. This sheet-like muscle lies beneath the other abdominal muscles and assists during many internal functions, such as coughing. It has little effect on abdominal appearance so we will not deal with it directly in this manual.

GETTING STARTED

Finally, here are a few practical considerations concerning the use of your Body Ball.

Ball Size

Your Body Ball should be large enough so that when you sit on it, your knees bend at a 90-degree angle.

Ball diameter is usually measured in centimeters. A person 5'0" to 5'7" would probably use a ball of approximately 55 cm; someone 5'8" or over would probably need one of 65 cm. (Balls of 45 and 75 cm are also available if your height falls greatly outside this range.) If in doubt, it's better to have a slightly larger Ball than one that's too small.

Inflation

Inflate the Ball to the point where it still "gives" but is firm enough to roll easily. The Ball will lose air pressure over time and will need to be repressurized every three months or so.

Cautions

- Keep your Ball away from all sources of heat.

- Do not wear jewelry or any sharp accessories while exercising.

- Do not use the Ball outdoors in direct sunlight or in temperatures warmer than 80 degrees F.

General Guidelines

- Perform all exercises slowly and deliberately.

- Follow the exercise descriptions carefully.

- Work into a movement gradually so that you get used to the pattern of the exercise and learn how to balance your body properly.

- If at any time you feel discomfort or pain, stop immediately and check your form — *severe discomfort should never accompany any exercise program.*

❖ ❖ ❖

That completes the basic information you should have under your belt before working out. In the next chapter, we'll cover the exercises that make up the *HFL Body Ball Routine.*

The Exercises

WARM-UPS

Although the *HFL Body Ball Routine* is non-impact and poses little risk of injury, it is still important to begin your exercise program with a five-to-10-minute warm-up. Warm-ups should be gradual, steadily increasing in tempo and effort until you reach the level of your upcoming workout. By the end of the warm-up, you should be sweating lightly.

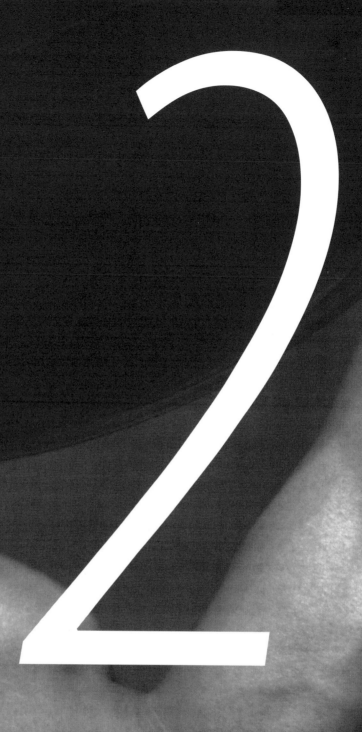

2

Giddyap

Purpose: This exercise will gently warm up your entire lower body; it will also help you improve your balance.

Begin by sitting on the Ball with your feet in front of you and your knees bent at 90-degree angles. With hands at your sides for stability, start bouncing by pushing off one foot at a time, while slightly lifting the opposite foot. Bounce for 60 seconds, working up to the optimum rate of 120 bounces per minute.

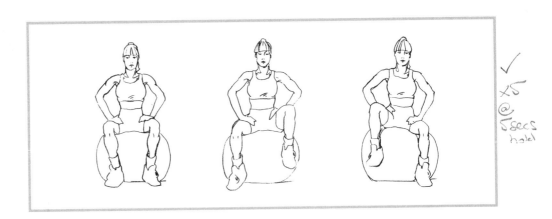

Ride Around the Ball

Purpose: General warm-up for the hip, leg, and lower abdominal muscles.

Begin by bouncing, this time pushing off both feet simultaneously. With each bounce, step to the side with one leg and follow with the other while pivoting on top of the Ball. Move only one leg per bounce. Walk a full circle clockwise, then repeat in the opposite direction.

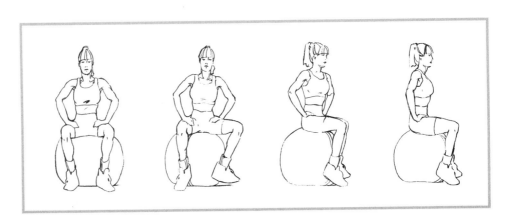

THE EXERCISES

Slalom

Purpose: General warm-up for the hip, leg, waist, and abdominal muscles. Builds muscular endurance in the front of the thighs while toning and tightening the waist.

Begin by bouncing on the Ball. Then, keeping your feet together, move them from side to side, alternating with each bounce like a slalom skier. Your hips and upper torso will naturally lean to the side that your feet are on; keep your elbows bent and swing your arms to the opposite side for balance, as though you were planting a ski pole with each bounce.

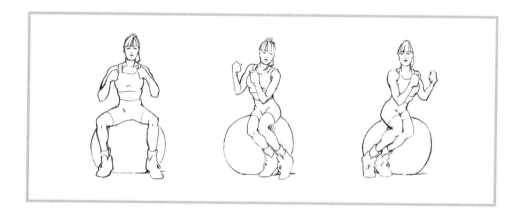

The Recliner

Purpose: Warm-up for the ankle, knee, leg, hip, and abdominal muscles.

Begin by sitting upright on the Ball with your hands on knees and your knees at a 90-degree angle. Walk forward, one leg at a time, allowing the Ball to roll upward along your spine to your upper back. Keep your torso rigid by elevating the hips and leaning back as you go. Continue to walk until the Ball reaches your shoulder blades.

Keep your head up throughout the movement. Return to upright position by reversing the motion: push with your legs so that the Ball rolls back down to the buttocks. Repeat.

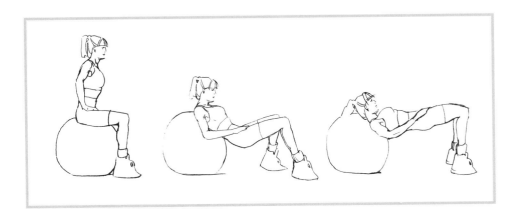

LOWER BODY

Wall Squats

Purpose: Tones and strengthens quadriceps, hamstrings, and buttock muscles.

If possible, use the corner of a room for greater stability while performing this exercise. If a corner is not available, any wall will do.

Standing with your back to the corner (or wall), adjust your feet so they are shoulder width apart, with toes pointing slightly outward. Place the Ball at the small of your back and lean against it, pressing it to the wall. Lower yourself into a squatting position to a count of four seconds down and four seconds up, emphasizing a slow and controlled movement. Focus on pushing off with your heels.

THE EXERCISES

Important: Place your feet far enough in front of your body that when you bend your knees and descend, your lower legs remain nearly vertical. Also, keep your pelvis tilted under, as shown in the *RIGHT* illustration below.

BEGINNING: QUARTER SQUATS

Descend only one-fourth of the possible distance and return.

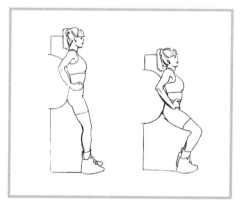

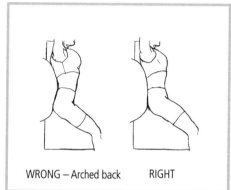
WRONG – Arched back   RIGHT

INTERMEDIATE: FULL SQUATS

Descend until your thighs are parallel to the floor and return. Once again, remember to place your feet far enough in front of your body that your lower legs remain nearly vertical when you squat.

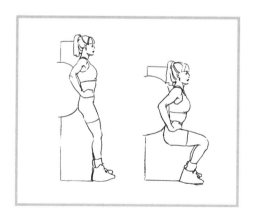

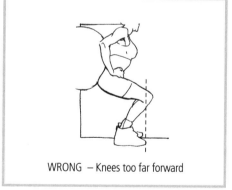
WRONG – Knees too far forward

1) Align feet + use the toes

2) Pelvic floor lift throughout

THE EXERCISES

ADVANCED: ONE-LEGGED SQUATS

Position the leg to be worked under the center of your body for balance and either rest the non-exercising leg on the working thigh or wrap it under the working leg. Hold on to a doorknob, chair or other fixed object for stability. Good luck—these are tough!

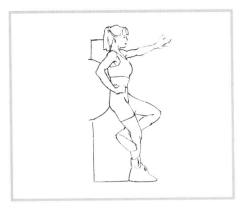 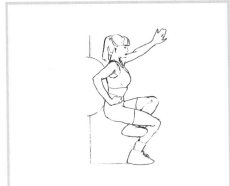

Wall Hack Squats

Purpose: Targets the front of the thighs just above the knees, as well as the buttocks and abdominals.

As with Wall Squats, using the corner of a room to perform this exercise will give you greater stability — but, again, any wall will do.

Standing with your back to the corner (or wall), adjust your feet so they are shoulder width apart, with your toes pointing slightly outward. Place the Ball at the small of your back and lean against it, pressing it to the wall. In this variation of Wall Squats, your feet should be placed far enough from the wall that your head and shoulders angle backward.

Begin to lower yourself into a squatting position. As you descend, raise your hips and squeeze your butt, maintaining an upward pelvic tilt. Lower into the bottom position to a count of four seconds, then ascend to a count of four seconds, emphasizing a slow and controlled movement. Focus on pushing with your heels.

BEGINNING: QUARTER HACK SQUATS

Descend only one-fourth of the possible distance and return.

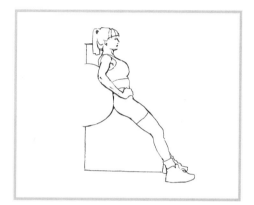
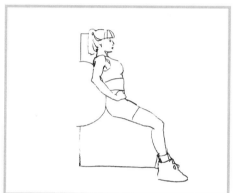

INTERMEDIATE: FULL HACK SQUATS

Descend until your thighs are parallel to the floor and return.

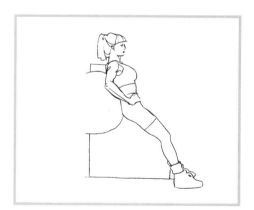
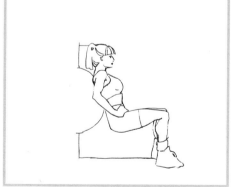

ADVANCED: ONE-LEGGED HACK SQUATS

Position the leg to be worked under the center of your body for balance. Rest the non-exercising leg on the working thigh or wrap it under the working leg. Hold on to a door knob, chair or other fixed object for stability.

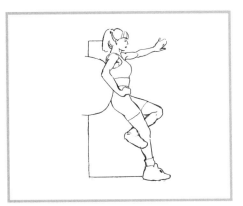
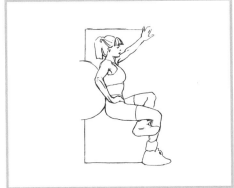

Hamstring Bridges

Purpose: Tones and strengthens the hamstrings.

Lie on your back with knees slightly bent and your heels and lower calves resting on the Ball. Your head should rest on the floor and your hands should be comfortably interlocked on your stomach. Raise your pelvis about five or six inches by squeezing the buttocks together and pressing through your heels into the Ball. Your knees will flex slightly. Feel the weight of your pelvis being supported by the backs of your legs. Lower and repeat.

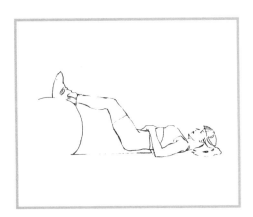
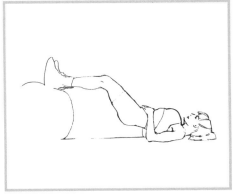

ADVANCED: ONE-LEGGED HAMSTRING BRIDGES

Place your working leg on the Ball as described above and hold your non-working leg in the air. Raise your pelvis by squeezing the buttocks together and pressing through your heel into the Ball. Your knee will flex slightly. Feel the weight of your pelvis being supported by the back of your leg. Switch legs and repeat.

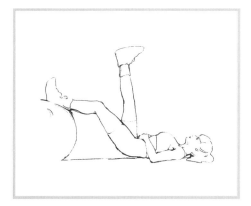 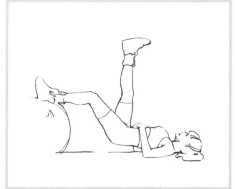

Glute Bridges

Purpose: Tones and strengthens buttocks and hamstrings.

Lie on your back with the Ball in close to your bottom. Rest only your heels on top of the Ball. Squeeze your buttocks together and raise your pelvis by pressing through your heels. Lower and repeat.

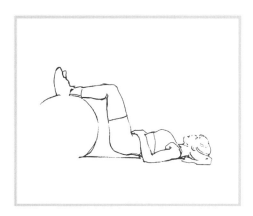 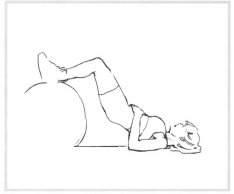

✓ 5 reps
@ 5 secs

ADVANCED: ONE-LEGGED GLUTE BRIDGES

Position your working leg on the Ball as described above but hold your non-working leg in the air. Squeeze your buttocks together and raise your pelvis by pressing through your heel. Switch legs and repeat.

Note: Until you develop the skill to do the exercise as described above, you can also stretch out your non-working leg on the floor, forming a curb against the Ball to keep it from rolling.

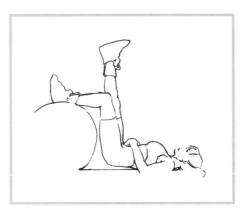 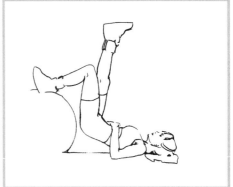

In-'n'-Out Rolls

Purpose: Tones and strengthens the glutes and hamstrings. Facilitates balance and muscle control.

Lie on the floor on your back, arms a few inches from your sides, palms down. (You can also rest your hands, interlocked comfortably, on your stomach.) Place your heels on the Ball, six inches apart for balance. Keeping your legs stiff and slightly bent at the knee, raise your pelvis until your body forms a straight line from your feet to your middle back (still resting on the floor). Now roll the Ball in until your knees are fully bent, maintaining pressure on the Ball with your heels, and maintaining a pelvic tilt and pelvic elevation at all times. Keep your neck relaxed and your head resting on the floor throughout the movement. Return the Ball to original position and repeat.

T H E   E X E R C I S E S

30

Note: As you draw the ball toward you, it will naturally roll upward along the soles of your feet, so that at the peak of the movement you will find yourself pushing through the balls of the feet, rather than the heels.

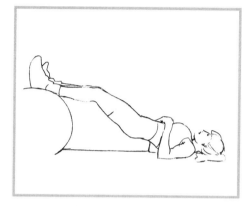

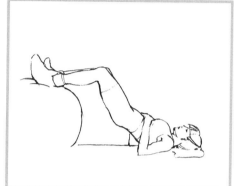

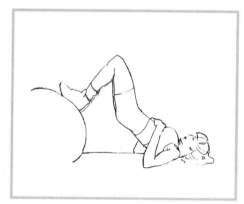

ADVANCED: ONE-LEGGED IN-'N'-OUT ROLLS

Begin in the same position but raise your non-working leg into the air while keeping your working heel at the top of the Ball. Elevate your pelvis and roll the Ball in and out as described above. Use your hands to stabilize yourself as needed.

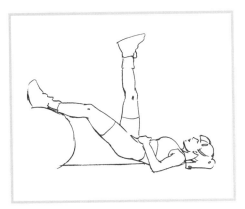 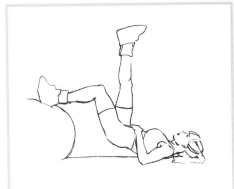

Dolphins

Purpose: Tones and strengthens the glutes, hamstrings, and spinal erectors.

Kneel, facing the Ball. Lean forward until your pelvis is supported by the Ball and your hands are on the floor supporting your upper body. Position yourself far enough forward to counterbalance the weight of your legs. Your feet should be together with your toes touching the floor. Keeping your legs slightly bent and stiff, raise them off the floor as high as you can, being sure to squeeze the buttocks and slightly arch the lower back. Lower your legs toward the floor (but don't touch!) and repeat.

THE EXERCISES

Note: A common mistake is to dip the head and torso with each rep. Be sure to keep your head forward and your arms straight.

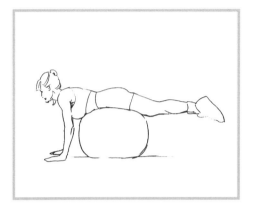 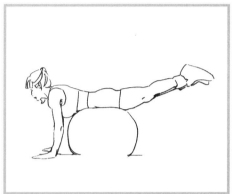

✓ 5 reps @
5 secs

Knee Squeezes

Purpose: Tones and strengthens the inner thigh muscles.

Sit on the floor in a butterfly position (i.e., a semi-lotus position, in which you match the soles of your feet together and flare your knees to the sides) and place the Ball between your knees and thighs. Squeeze your knees together slowly and carefully just a few inches. Hold for one full second, then slowly release toward the starting position, always maintaining the tension in your inner thighs. Repeat.

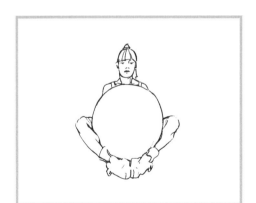 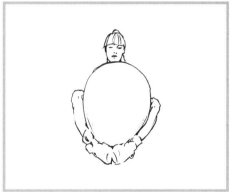

ADVANCED: UPRIGHT KNEE SQUEEZES

Sit on the Ball with your feet behind you and your toes touching the floor. Your knees should point downward. Squeeze your knees together so that your whole body elevates with each squeeze. Hold each squeeze for one second and release slowly so that you maintain the tension in your inner thighs throughout the motion. Repeat.

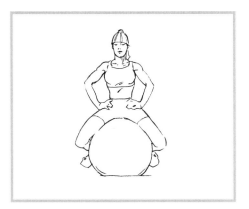 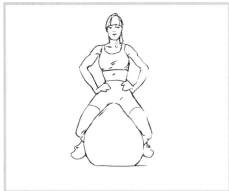

Leaning Inner-Thigh Lifts

Purpose: Tones and strengthens the inner thigh muscles.

Lean sideways on the Ball, holding it underneath your arm. Plant your hand on the floor for balance. Your lower leg should be outstretched while the other is bent to help you stay in position. Raise the foot of your lower leg about 12 inches off the floor, rotating your leg so that as you lift, your foot remains parallel to the floor. Do not touch the floor between repetitions. Repeat on the other side.

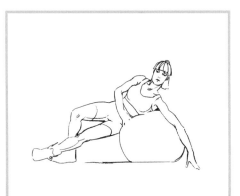 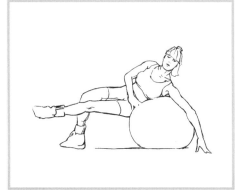

34

Side Kicks

Purpose: Tones and strengthens the hip and buttock muscles.

Kneel on one knee and place the Ball directly to the outside of the weight-bearing leg. Lean sideways onto the Ball so that it supports your waist, placing one hand on the Ball and one hand on the floor for balance. Stretch your free leg straight out to the side and hold it rigid. Maintain a strict sideways position to the Ball at all times. Raise your leg as high as possible, pointing your toe sightly toward the floor (internally rotating at the hip). Squeeze the buttocks with each repetition. Repeat.

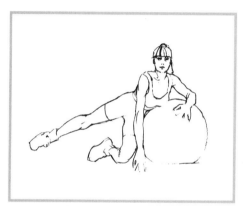
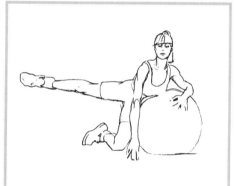
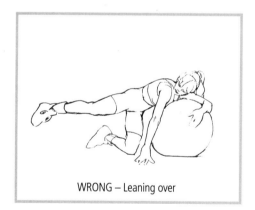

WRONG – Leaning over

Leaning Calf Raises

Purpose: Tones, strengthens, and stretches the calf muscles.

Stand facing the wall. Place the Ball between your chest and the wall, leaning forward to hold it in place. Adjust the distance of your feet from the wall until they are as far away as possible but still comfortably flat on the floor. (You should feel a calf stretch in this position.) Place your hands on top of the Ball for balance. Rise as high as possible onto the balls of your feet, then slowly lower yourself until your heels touch the floor.

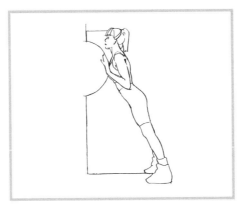 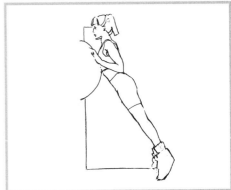

ADVANCED: ONE-LEGGED CALF RAISES

The one-legged version is the same as described above, except that you center your working leg below you for better balance and rest your free leg on the calf muscle of the working leg. Rise as high as possible onto the ball of your foot, then slowly lower yourself until your heel touches the floor. Repeat.

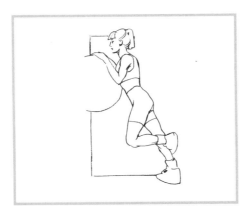 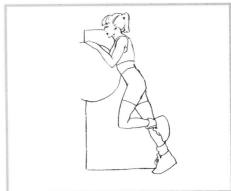

CHAPTER 2

LOWER BACK

Supermans

Purpose: Tones the back, buttocks and leg muscles. Improves coordination and balance.

Drape your body over the Ball so that it supports your midsection. Place your feet close together with toes touching the floor. Raise one arm and its opposite leg simultaneously, keeping both straight as you do so and allowing your back to extend and arch slightly. Maintain a slow, gentle pace, alternating arms and legs with each repetition.

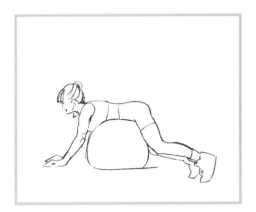
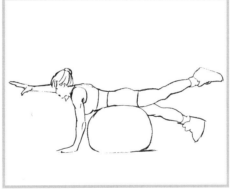

Hyperextensions

Purpose: Tones and strengthens the back and buttock muscles.

Drape your body over the Ball so that it supports your midsection. Your feet should be shoulder width apart, your toes firmly braced against a wall or large piece of furniture for stability. Place your hands behind your head and lower your torso until your elbows touch the floor. Keep your back rounded, following the curve of the Ball. Now raise your upper body one segment at a time: Begin by raising head and elbows, then upper back, and finally lower back, until your torso is arched upwards in a "swan dive" position. Lower and repeat.

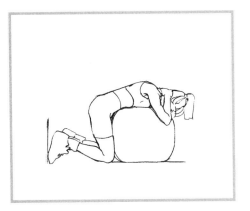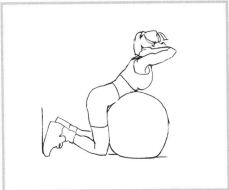

ABDOMINALS

Pelvic Tilts

Purpose: Tones and strengthens the abdominal muscles.

Beginning from a seated position on the Ball, walk your feet forward, allowing the ball to roll up under your lower back. Clasp your hands behind your head, and, keeping your neck and shoulders rounded, use your lower abs to tilt your pelvis upward as you perform a crunch with your upper abdominals. Do not let your back arch between reps.

Visualize your abdominal muscles contracting like an accordion, and remember that the range of motion for ab contraction is only 30 degrees. Hold in the contracted position for five seconds. Repeat.

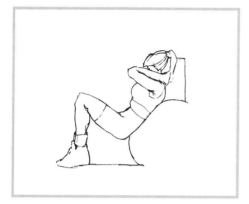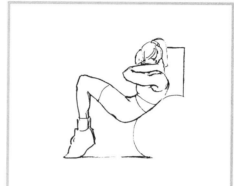

Lying Leg Thrusts

Purpose: Tones and strengthens the abdominal muscles, specifically targeting the lower portion of the abs.

Lie on your back, holding the Ball by squeezing it firmly between your calves and ankles. Place your fists palms down beneath your pelvis on either side of your tailbone. This should cause your pelvis to tip up toward your stomach, flattening your lower spine against the ground. Make sure your lower back is flat on the floor at the start of the exercise. Adjust your hand position to prevent your back from arching.

With fists supporting hips, raise your head — and shoulders, if possible — slightly off the ground. Now raise your legs and the Ball about 14 to 18 inches off the floor — high enough so that you can feel your lower back press against the floor. Bending at the waist (not the hips), raise your legs and pelvis until your feet point straight up. Then thrust upward from your pelvis as though trying to press the Ball against the ceiling. (Be careful to maintain your grip on the ball at this point or it may drop on your face!) Then drop straight down, retracing the upward path and allowing your legs to return to the starting position 14 to 18 inches off the floor. Repeat.

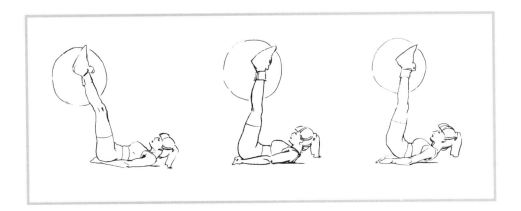

Crunches

Purpose: Tones and strengthens the upper abdominal muscles.

Lie on your back with your knees bent at a 90-degree angle, heels resting on the Ball. Place your hands behind your head to support your neck. Slowly raise your shoulders and upper back about 30 degrees off the ground, focusing on raising your torso upward to the ceiling, rather than to your knees. Hold the contraction for one second and return to the starting position. Repeat.

Note: Your hands should merely support your head — do not pull on your neck.

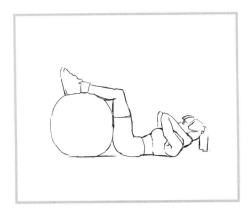 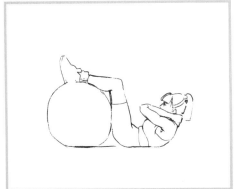

THE EXERCISES

Cross Crunches

Purpose: Tones and strengthens the upper abdominal and oblique muscles.

Lie on your back with your knees bent and your feet flat on the floor. Rest the Ball on to your abdomen, holding it with hands about shoulder width apart. Raise your head and shoulders and tuck your chin to your chest. Begin by raising your right shoulder and pushing with your right hand. This will move the Ball up your left thigh to the top of your left knee, emphasizing the rotation of your torso and contraction of your abdominals. Avoid using arms and shoulders in place of this torso rotation. Drop the Ball, retracing your upward path. Repeat on the right side.

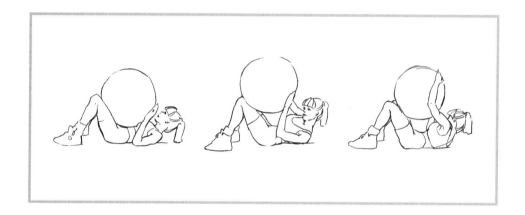

Springboards

Purpose: Tones and strengthens the ab muscles. Improves balance and coordination.

Stretch out in a stiff, prone position, balancing on the Ball on your upper thigh and hip area. Extend your arms, bracing your hands on the floor to steady yourself. Your head, spine, and legs should form a straight line. Keeping your arms extended, bend your knees and curl up into a fetal position, allowing the Ball to roll toward your chest. As you do so, make sure to round your back, tuck in your head, and bring your knees close to your head. Reverse the motion and return to the starting position.

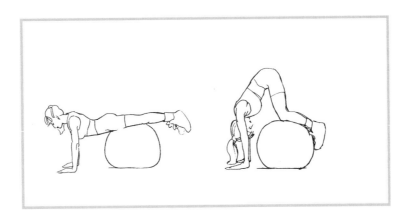

STRETCHES

After the toning portion of your workout, your muscles will be warm and elastic. This is the best time to do flexibility exercises. When your muscles are warm, you can stretch further with greater safety and ease.

Important Performance Point: Enter all stretching movements slowly and steadily, hold — without bouncing — for 10 to 15 seconds, and then carefully release and return to the starting position.

Back Roll

Purpose: Stretches the spine, abs, and chest muscles.

Lie backward over the Ball with arms extended, being careful to support your head on the Ball. Your knees should be bent at a 90-degree angle. Push with your feet, rolling yourself "upward" over the Ball so that your arms and head move toward the floor. Reach with your arms. Hold for 30 seconds and repeat.

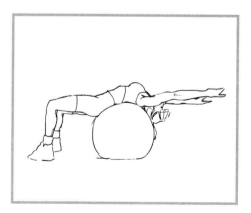

T H E   E X E R C I S E S

Side Stretch

Purpose: Stretches the lats, pecs, and oblique muscles.

Kneel on one knee, placing the Ball directly to the outside of the weight-bearing leg. Lean sideways onto the Ball so that it supports you at the waist. Extend your legs in a scissor position. Lower your head onto the shoulder that is against the Ball and lift your free arm over your head. Relax and hold for 30 seconds. Repeat.

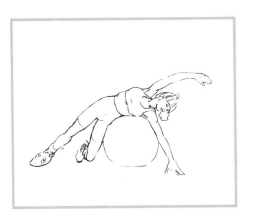

Hamstring Stretch

Purpose: Stretches the hamstring and calf muscles.

Kneel on one knee, resting the calf of the other on the Ball in front of you. Reach forward, grasp your toes and gently pull them toward you, keeping your knee straight or very slightly bent. Slowly bend your torso forward. Hold for 30 seconds and repeat.

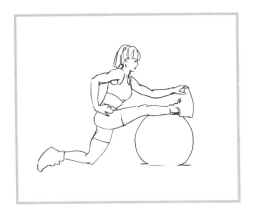

C H A P T E R

2

Straddler Stretch

Purpose: Stretches the hip flexor muscles.

Assume a lunging stance with the Ball tucked in close to the front of your weight-bearing knee. Lean forward, resting your pelvic area on the Ball, shifting your weight onto it

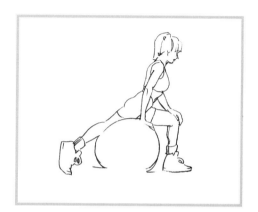

while extending your rear leg as far back as possible. Roll forward on the Ball, feeling a stretch in the top of the thigh.

The Swan

Purpose: Stretches the buttocks, hip and back muscles.

Assume a half-kneeling stance and place the Ball in front of your forward knee. Rest your hands on top of the Ball to steady yourself, and cross your front leg over your rear leg. Bend forward and extend your rear leg, feeling a stretch in the hip. Use the Ball for support, keeping it as far in front of you as possible for maximum stretch. Hold for 30 seconds and repeat with the other leg.

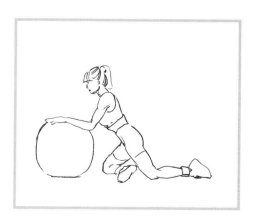
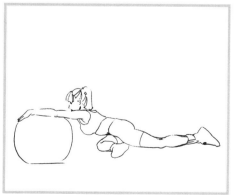

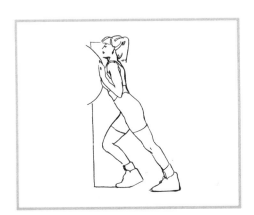

Ball Splits

Purpose: Stretches the inner thigh muscles.

Kneel on one knee, holding the other leg to the side and resting it on the ball. (Hold onto a chair or other support to maintain balance.) Slowly and gently lean toward the ball, allowing it to roll away from your supporting leg. Feel a stretch in the inner thigh. Maintain forward pelvic tilt. Hold for 30 seconds and repeat with the other leg.

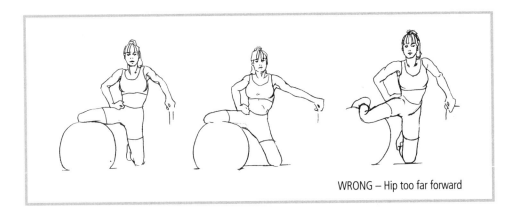

WRONG – Hip too far forward

Leaning Calf Stretch

Purpose: Stretches the calf muscles.

Stand, facing the wall. Place the Ball between your chest and the wall, leaning forward to hold it in place. Place one foot 12 to 18 inches in front of the other, and adjust your distance from the wall to feel a stretch in your rear leg while keeping your rear foot flat on the ground. Keep your hands on top of the Ball for balance. Hold for 30 seconds. Switch feet and repeat.

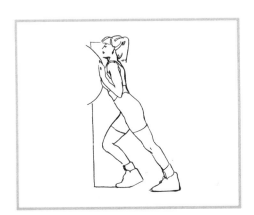

THE EXERCISES

The Body Ball Routine

ROUTINE BASICS

In this chapter, we'll take the exercises illustrated in *Chapter 2* and combine them to form the *HFL Body Ball Routine*. The routine has five levels, ranging from easy to difficult. Each level consists of four sections —*Warm-up*, *Exercises*, *Abdominals*, and *Stretches*. The *Stretches* section is the same for all levels but is repeated on each so you don't have to flip back through the book once you've advanced beyond *Level 1*.

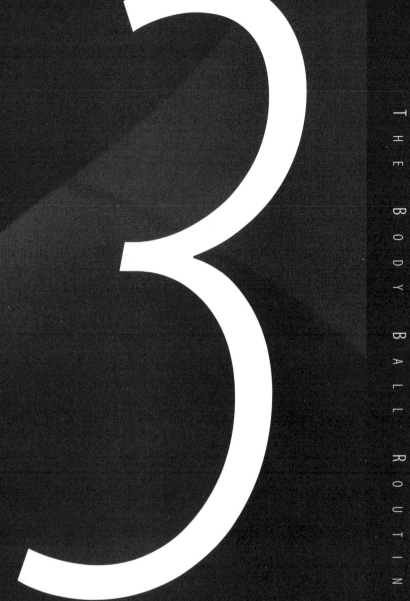

3

THE BODY BALL ROUTINE

Rest

The amount of rest you should allow varies from level to level. Follow the guidelines at the head of each section. Pay particular attention to the fact that some of the notes concern rest between *sets*, while others concern rest between *exercises*.

Supersets

The higher levels of the *Body Ball Routine* make use of supersets. A superset is two exercises performed back-to-back without rest. In the routines, a superset is indicated like this...

2 supersets	**Hamstring Bridges** (Beg.)	15–20 reps
	Wall Squats (Int.)	15–20 reps

To perform these two supersets, you would:

• Do a set of Hamstring Bridges followed immediately by a set of Wall Squats (that's the first superset).

• Rest for the amount of time listed at the beginning of the workout section for *Rest Between Sets.*

• Do another set of Hamstring Bridges followed immediately by another set of Wall Squats (that's the second superset).

If the note "(each leg)" or "(each side)" appears after the name of an exercise within the superset, like this...

2 supersets	**Supermans**	10 reps (each side)
	Hyperextensions	15–20 reps

...it means one of the exercises in the superset is a single-leg movement. Here, you would do two sets of the first exercise — one for each leg — plus a set of the second exercise before starting the next superset (e.g. Exercise A, left leg; Exercise A, right leg; Exercise B; Exercise A, left leg; Exercise A, right leg; Exercise B; and so on).

Giant Sets

Level 5 uses **giant sets** as well as supersets. A giant set is just like a superset, except, instead of being two exercises performed back-to-back without rest, it's *three or more* exercises performed back-to-back without rest.

3 giant sets	**Dolphins**	15 reps
	Glute Bridges (Beg.)	20 reps
	Wall Squats (Int.)	20 reps

Level 5 calls for 3 giant sets of Dolphins, Glute Bridges, and Wall Squats. ***To perform these three giant sets, you would:***

- Do a set of Dolphins, followed immediately by a set of Glute Bridges, followed immediately by a set of Wall Squats (that's the first giant set).

- Rest for the amount of time listed at the beginning of the workout section for *Rest Between Sets*.

- Repeat the whole cycle twice more.

Illustrated Routine

The routine appears first in written form, beginning on the next page, then in graphic form, beginning on page 62.

Level 1

WARM-UP NO REST BETWEEN EXERCISES

1 set	**Giddyap**	25 bounces
1 set	**Ride Around the Ball**	1 revolution, right 1 revolution, left

EXERCISES 30 SEC REST BETWEEN SETS AND EXERCISES

3 sets	**Wall Squats - 1/4 Squat** (Beg.)	10-15 reps
2 sets	**Hamstring Bridges** (Beg.)	6–10 reps
2 sets	**In-'n'-Out Rolls** (Beg.)	15–20 reps
1 set	**Dolphins**	8–10 reps
2 sets	**Knee Squeezes** (Beg.)	10–12 reps
2 sets	**Side Kicks**	15–20 reps (each leg)
2 sets	**Leaning Calf Raises** (Beg.)	15–20 reps
1 set	**Supermans**	10 reps (each side)

CHAPTER 3

ABS   30 SEC REST BETWEEN EXERCISES

1 set	**Pelvic Tilts**	12–15 reps
1 set	**Crunches**	15–20 reps

STRETCHES   NO REST BETWEEN EXERCISES

1 rep	**Back Roll**	15–20 secs
1 rep	**Side Stretch**	15–20 secs (each side)
1 rep	**Hamstring Stretch**	15–20 secs (each leg)
1 rep	**Swan**	15–20 secs (each hip)
1 rep	**Leaning Calf Stretch**	15–20 secs (each leg)

Level 2

WARM-UP NO REST BETWEEN EXERCISES

1 set	**Giddyap**	50 bounces
1 set	**Ride Around the Ball**	2 revolutions, right 2 revolutions, left

EXERCISES 30 SEC REST BETWEEN SETS AND EXERCISES

2 sets	**Wall Hack Squats – 1/4** (Beg.)	10–15 reps
2 sets	**Wall Squats** (Int.)	10–15 reps
1 set	**Hamstring Bridges** (Beg.)	10–15 reps (each leg)
3 sets	**In-'n'-Out Rolls** (Beg.)	15–20 reps
2 sets	**Dolphins**	20 reps
3 sets	**Knee Squeezes** (Beg.)	10–12 reps
2 sets	**Side Kicks**	15–20 reps (each leg)
3 sets	**Leaning Calf Raises** (Adv.)	15–20 reps
2 sets	**Supermans**	10 reps (each side)

54

ABS   30 SEC REST BETWEEN SETS AND EXERCISES

1 set	**Lying Leg Thrusts**	12-15 reps
2 sets	**Crunches**	15–20 reps
1 set	**Cross Crunches**	15 reps (each side)

STRETCHES   NO REST BETWEEN EXERCISES

1 rep	**Back Roll**	15–20 secs
1 rep	**Side Stretch**	15–20 secs (each side)
1 rep	**Hamstring Stretch**	15–20 secs (each leg)
1 rep	**Swan**	15–20 secs (each hip)
1 rep	**Leaning Calf Stretch**	15–20 secs (each leg)

THE BODY BALL ROUTINE

Level 3

WARM-UP NO REST BETWEEN EXERCISES

1 set	**Giddyap**	90 secs @ 120 bounces/min.
1 set	**Ride Around The Ball**	2 revolutions, right 2 revolutions, left
1 set	**Slalom**	30 bounces (each side)

EXERCISES 30 SEC REST BETWEEN SETS AND EXERCISES

3 sets	**Wall Hack Squats** (Int.)	15–20 reps
2 sets	**Wall Squats** (Int.)	15–20 reps
2 sets	**Hamstrings Bridges** (Beg.)	10–15 reps
1 set	**Glute Bridges** (Beg.)	10–15 reps
2 sets	**In-'n'-Out Rolls** (Beg.)	15–20 (each side)
2 sets	**Dolphins**	20 reps
3 sets	**Knee Squeezes** (Adv.)	10–15 reps
2 sets	**Leaning Inner-Thigh Raises**	20 reps (each leg)
2 sets	**Side Kicks**	15–20 reps (each side)
2 sets	**Leaning Calf Raises** (Adv.)	15–20 reps (each leg)
2 sets	**Hyperextensions**	10–15 reps

ABS   15 SEC REST BTWN SETS; NO REST BTWN EXERCISES

2 sets	**Lying Leg Thrusts**	12–15 reps
2 sets	**Crunches**	25 reps
1 set	**Cross Crunches**	25 reps (each side)

STRETCHES   NO REST BETWEEN EXERCISES

1 rep	**Back Roll**	15–20 secs
1 rep	**Side Stretch**	15–20 secs (each side)
1 rep	**Hamstring Stretch**	15–20 secs (each leg)
1 rep	**Swan**	15–20 secs (each hip)
1 rep	**Leaning Calf Stretch**	15–20 secs (each leg)

Level 4

WARM-UP   NO REST BETWEEN EXERCISES

1 set	**Giddyap**	3 min. @ 120 bounces/min.
1 set	**Ride Around The Ball**	3 revolutions, right 3 revolutions, left
1 set	**Slalom**	90 secs. @ 120 bounces/min
1 set	**Recliner**	10 reps

EXERCISES   15 SEC REST BTWN SETS; NO REST BTWN EXERCISES

1 set	**Wall Hack Squats** (Adv.)	10–15 reps (each side)
3 sets	**Glute Bridges** (Beg.)	15–20 reps
2 supersets	**Hamstring Bridges** (Beg.) **Wall Squats** (Int.)	15–20 reps 15–20 reps
2 sets	**In-'n'-Out Rolls** (Adv.)	15–20 reps (each side)
2 sets	**Leaning Inner-Thigh Raises**	20 reps (each leg)
3 sets	**Knee Squeezes** (Adv.)	15–20 reps
2 sets	**Side Kicks**	30 reps
3 sets	**Leaning Calf Raises** (Adv.)	15–20 reps
2 supersets	**Supermans** **Hyperextensions**	10 reps (each side) 15–20 reps

ABS 10 SEC REST BETWEEN EXERCISES

1 set	**Lying Leg Thrusts**	20 reps
1 superset	**Lying Leg Thrusts** **Crunches**	15 reps 25 reps
1 superset	**Cross Crunches** **Crunches**	20 reps 20 reps
1 set	**Springboards**	15–20 reps

STRETCHES   NO REST BETWEEN EXERCISES

1 rep	**Back Roll**	15–20 secs
1 rep	**Side Stretch**	15–20 secs (each side)
1 rep	**Hamstring Stretch**	15–20 secs (each leg)
1 rep	**Swan**	15–20 secs (each hip)
1 rep	**Leaning Calf Stretch**	15–20 secs (each leg)

THE BODY BALL ROUTINE

Level 5

WARM-UP   NO REST BETWEEN EXERCISES

1 set	**Giddyap**	3–5 min. @ 120 bounces/min.
1 set	**Ride Around the Ball**	5 Revolutions, right 5 Revolutions, left
1 set	**Slalom**	1–3 min. @ 120 bounces/min.
1 set	**Recliner**	15 reps

EXERCISES   10 SEC REST BTWN SETS; NO REST BTWN EXERCISES

3 sets	**Wall Hack Squats** (Adv.)	20–25 reps (each side)
2 supersets	**Hamstring Bridges** (Adv.) **In-'n'-Out Rolls** (Adv.)	20 reps (each leg) 20 reps (each leg)
1 set	**Glute Bridges** (Beg.)	20 reps
3 giant sets	**Dolphins** **Glute Bridges** (Beg.) **Wall Squats** (Int.)	15 reps 20 reps 15 reps (each leg)
3 sets	**Leaning Inner-Thigh Raises**	20 reps (each leg)
3 sets	**Knee Squeezes** (Adv.)	20–25 reps
3 sets	**Side Kicks**	25 reps (each leg)
3 sets	**Leaning Calf Raises** (Adv.)	25–30 reps (each leg)

3 supersets	**Supermans**	15 reps (each side)
	Hyperextensions	20–25 reps

ABS NO REST BETWEEN SETS OR EXERCISES

2 supersets	**Lying Leg Thrusts**	20 reps
	Crunches	35 reps
2 supersets	**Cross Crunches**	30 reps
	Crunches	35 reps
2 sets	**Springboards**	30 reps

STRETCHES NO REST BETWEEN EXERCISES

1 rep	**Back Roll**	15–20 secs
1 rep	**Side Stretch**	15–20 secs (each side)
1 rep	**Hamstring Stretch**	15–20 secs (each leg)
1 rep	**Swan**	15–20 secs (each hip)
1 rep	**Leaning Calf Stretch**	15–20 secs (each leg)

Body Ball Routine

Level 1

Giddyap
1 Set / 25 Bounces / pg 22

Ride Around the Ball
1 Revolution, Right / pg 22

Ride Around the Ball
1 Revolution, Left / pg 22

WARM UP

NO REST BETWEEN EXERCISES

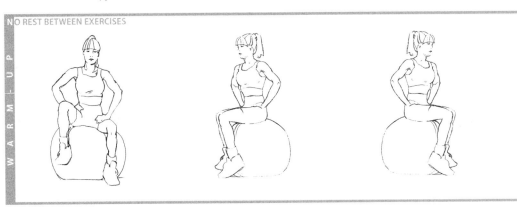

Dolphins
1 Sets / 8-10 Reps / pg 32

Knee Squeezes (Beg.)
2 Sets / 10-12 Reps / pg 33

Side Kicks
2 Sets / 15-20 Reps (ea. leg) / pg 35

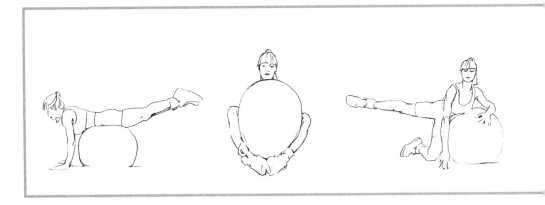

Wall Squats - 1/4 (Beg.)
3 Sets / 10-15 Reps / pg 25

Hamstring Bridges (Beg.)
2 Sets / 6-10 Reps / pg 28

In-'n'- Out Rolls (Beg.)
2 Set / 15-20 Reps / pg 30

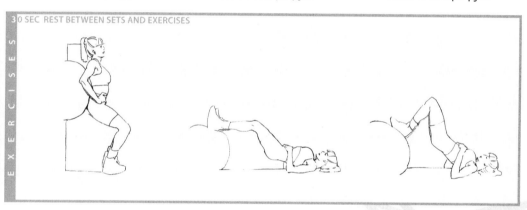

30 SEC REST BETWEEN SETS AND EXERCISES

EXERCISES

Leaning Calf Raises (Beg.)
2 Sets / 15-20 Reps / pg 36

Supermans
1 Set / 10 Reps (ea. side) / pg 37

Pelvic Tilts
1 Set / 12-15 Reps / pg 38

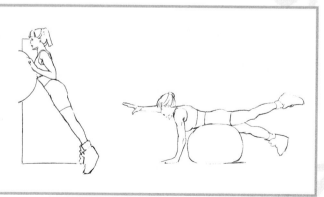

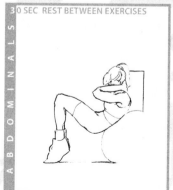

30 SEC REST BETWEEN EXERCISES

ABDOMINALS

Crunches
1 Set / 15-20 Reps / pg 40

Back Roll
1 Rep / 15-20 Seconds / pg 43

Side Stretch
1 Rep / 15-20 Sec (ea. side) / pg 44

NO REST BETWEEN EXERCISES

S T R E T C H E S

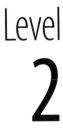

Giddyap
1 Set / 50 Bounces / pg 22

Ride Around the Ball
1 Set / 2 Revolutions, Right / pg 22

Ride Around the Ball
1 Set / 2 Revolutions, Left / pg 22

Level
2

NO REST BETWEEN EXERCISES

W A R M - U P

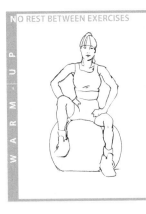

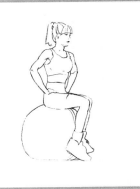

In-'n'- Out Rolls (Beg.)
3 Sets / 15-20 Reps / pg 30

Dolphins
2 Sets / 20 Reps / pg 32

Knee Squeezes (Beg.)
3 Sets / 10-12 Reps / pg 33

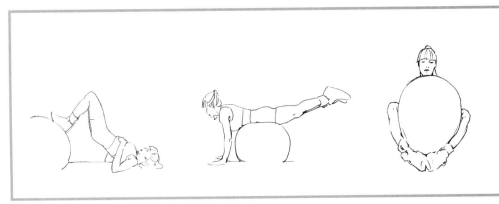

Hamstring Stretch
1 Rep / 15-20 Sec (ea. leg) / pg 44

Swan
1 Rep / 15-20 Sec (ea. hip) / pg 45

Leaning Calf Stretch
1 Rep / 15-20 Sec (ea. leg) / pg 46

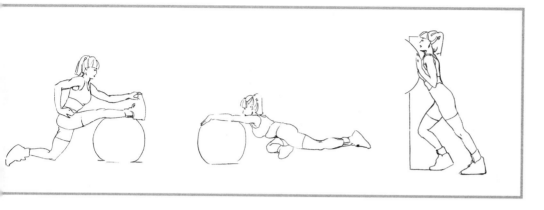

Wall Hack Squats – 1/4 (Beg.)
2 Sets / 10-15 Reps / pg 27

Wall Squats (Int.)
2 Sets / 10-15 Reps / pg 25

Hamstring Bridges (Beg.)
1 Set / 10-15 Reps (ea. leg) / pg 28

30 SEC REST BETWEEN SETS AND EXERCISES

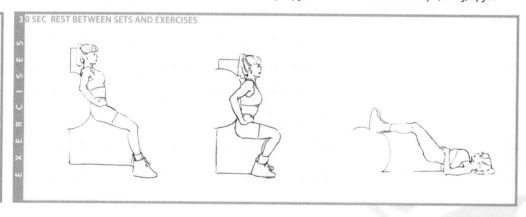

Side Kicks
2 Sets / 15-20 Reps (ea. leg) / pg 35

Leaning Calf Raises (Beg.)
3 Sets / 15-20 Reps / pg 36

Supermans
2 Sets / 10 Reps (ea. side) / pg 37

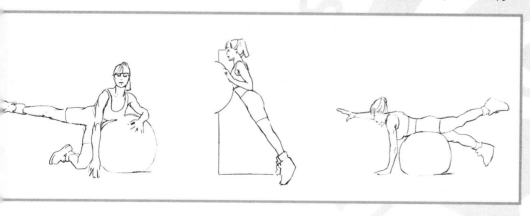

Lying Leg Thrusts
1 Set / 12-15 Reps / pg 39

Crunches
2 Sets / 15-20 Reps / pg 40

Cross Crunches
1 Set / 15 Reps (ea. side) / pg 41

30 SEC REST BETWEEN SETS; NO REST BETWEEN EXERCISES

ABDOMINALS

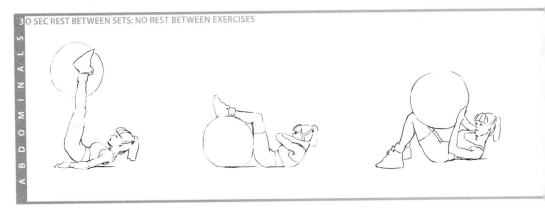

Swan
1 Rep / 15-20 Sec (ea. hip) / pg 45

Leaning Calf Stretch
1 Rep / 15-20 Sec (ea. leg) / pg 46

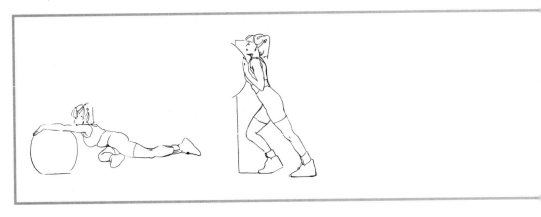

Giddyap
1 Set / 90 sec @ 120 Bncs/Min / pg 22

Ride Around the Ball
1 Set / 2 Revolutions, Right / pg 22

Ride Around the Ball
1 Set / 2 Revolutions, Left / pg 22

Level
3

NO REST BETWEEN EXERCISES

WARM-UP

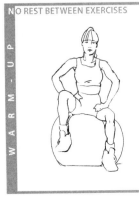
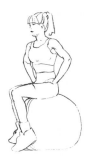
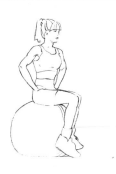

Back Roll
1 Rep / 15-20 Sec / pg 43

Side Stretch
1 Rep / 15-20 Sec (ea. side) / pg 44

Hamstring Stretch
1 Rep / 15-20 Sec (ea. leg) / pg 44

NO REST BETWEEN EXERCISES

STRETCHES

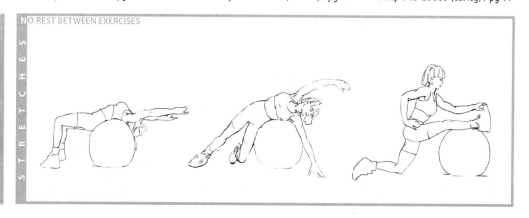

Slalom
1 Set / 30 Bncs (ea. side) / pg 23

Wall Hack Squats (Int.)
3 Sets / 15-20 Reps / pg 27

Wall Squats (Int.)
2 Sets / 15-20 Reps / pg 25

30 SEC REST BETWEEN SETS AND EXERCISES

EXERCISES

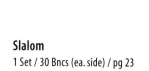

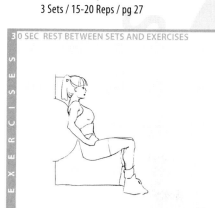

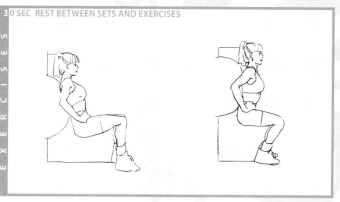

Hamstring Bridges (Beg.)
2 Set / 10-15 Reps / pg 28

Glute Bridges (Beg.)
1 Set / 10-15 Reps / pg 29

In-'n'-Out Rolls (Beg.)
2 Sets / 15-20 Reps (ea. side) / pg 30

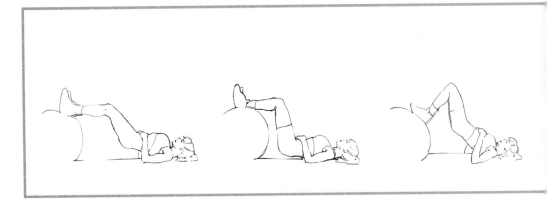

Side Kicks
2 Sets / 15-20 Reps (ea. leg) / pg 35

Leaning Calf Raises (Adv.)
2 Sets / 15-20 Reps (ea. leg) / pg 36

Hyperextensions
2 Sets / 10-15 Reps / pg 37

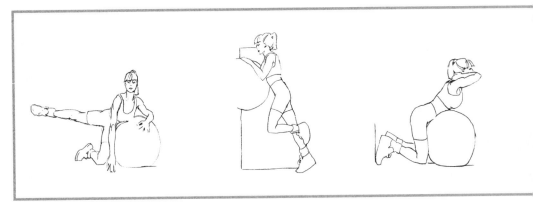

Back Roll
1 Rep / 15-20 Sec / pg 43

Side Stretch
1 Rep / 15-20 Sec (ea. side) / pg 44

Hamstring Stretch
1 Rep / 15-20 Sec (ea. leg) / pg 44

NO REST BETWEEN EXERCISES

STRETCHES

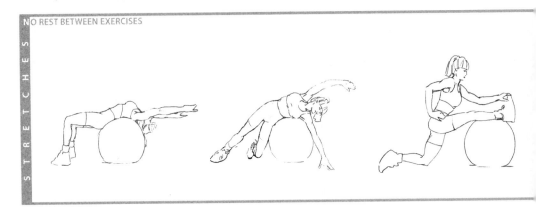

Dolphins
2 Sets / 20 Reps / pg 32

Knee Squeezes (Adv.)
3 Sets / 10-15 Reps / pg 34

Leaning Inner-Thigh Lifts
2 Sets / 20 Reps (ea. leg) / pg 34

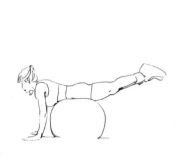 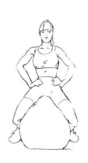 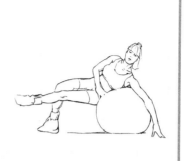

Lying Leg Thrusts
2 Sets / 12-15 Reps / pg 39

Crunches
2 Sets / 25 Reps / pg 40

Cross Crunches
1 Set / 25 Reps (ea. side) / pg 41

ABDOMINALS

15 SEC REST BETWEEN SETS; NO REST BETWEEN EXERCISES

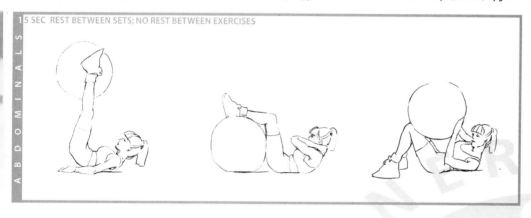

Swan
1 Rep / 15-20 Sec (ea. hip) / pg 45

Leaning Calf Stretch
1 Rep / 15-20 Sec (ea. leg) / pg 46

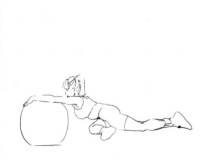 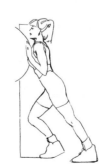

Level
4

WARM-UP

Giddyap
1 Set / 3 min @ 120 Bncs/min / pg 22

Ride Around the Ball
1 Set / 3 Revolutions, Right / pg 22

Ride Around the Ball
1 Set / 3 Revolutions, Left / pg 22

NO REST BETWEEN EXERCISES

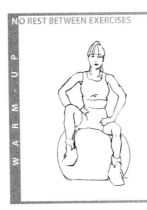
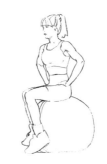
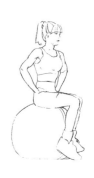

Glute Bridges (Beg.)
3 Sets / 15-20 Reps / pg 29

Hamstring Bridges (Beg.)
15-20 Reps / pg 28

Wall Squats (Int.)
15-20 Reps / pg 25

NO REST BETWEEN EXERCISES

2 SUPERSETS

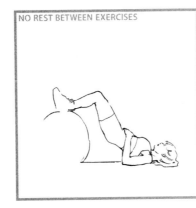
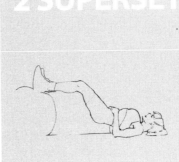
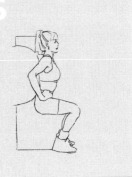

Side Kicks
2 Sets / 30 Reps (ea. leg) / pg 35

Leaning Calf Raises (Adv.)
3 Sets / 15-20 Reps (ea. leg) / pg 36

Supermans
10 Reps (ea. side) / pg 37

2 SUPERSETS

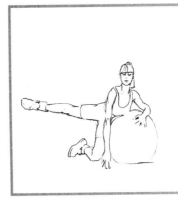
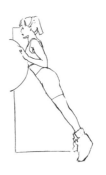
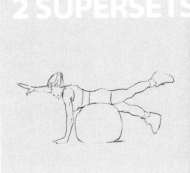

Slalom
1 Set / 90 Sec @ 120 Bncs/Min / pg 23

Recliner
1 Set / 10 Reps / pg 23

Wall Hack Squats (Adv.)
1 Set / 10-15 Reps (ea. side) / pg 28

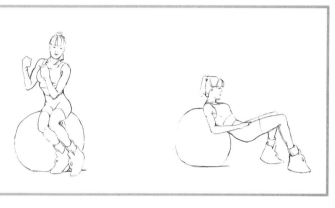

15 SEC REST BETWEEN SETS;

EXERCISES

In-'n'- Out Rolls (Adv.)
2 Set / 15-20 Reps (ea. side) / pg 32

Leaning Inner Thigh Lifts
2 Sets / 20 Reps (ea. leg) / pg 34

Knee Squeezes (Adv.)
3 Sets / 15-20 Reps / pg 34

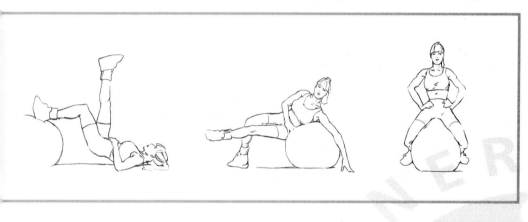

Hyperextensions
15-20 Reps / pg 37

Lying Leg Thrusts
1 Set / 20 Reps / pg 39

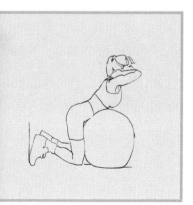

10 SEC REST BETWEEN EXERCISES (EXCEPT WITHIN SUPERSETS)

ABDOMINALS

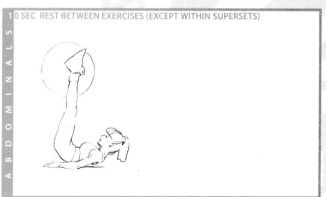

| **Lying Leg Thrusts**
15 Reps / pg 39 | **Crunches**
25 Reps / pg 40 | **Cross Crunches**
20 Reps / pg 41 |

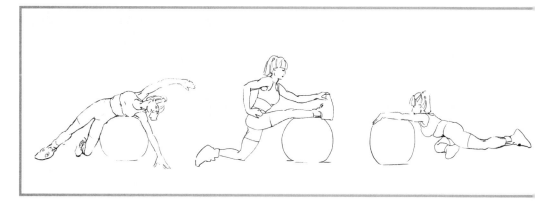

1 SUPERSET   **1 SUPERSET**

| **Side Stretch**
1 Rep / 10-15 Sec (ea. side) / pg 44 | **Hamstring Stretch**
1 Rep / 10-15 Sec (ea. leg) / pg 44 | **Swan**
1 Rep / 15-20 Sec (ea. hip) / pg 45 |

| **Giddyap**
1 Set / 3-5 Min @ 120 Bncs/Min / pg 22 | **Ride Around the Ball**
1 Set / 5 Revolutions, Right / pg 22 | **Ride Around the Ball**
1 Set / 5 Revolutions, Left / pg 22 |

Level
5

NO REST BETWEEN EXERCISES

W A R M - U P

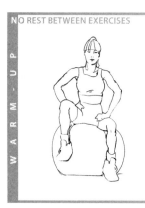
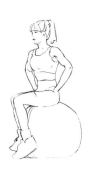
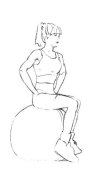

Crunches
20 Reps / pg 40

Springboards
1 Set / 15-20 Reps / pg 42

Back Roll
1 Rep / 15-20 Sec / pg 43

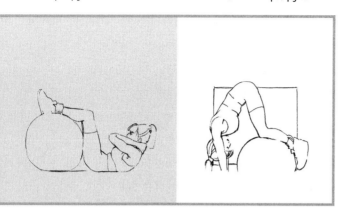

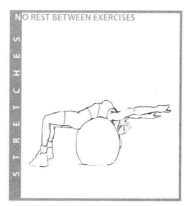

NO REST BETWEEN EXERCISES

S T R E T C H E S

Leaning Calf Stretch
1 Rep / 15-20 Sec (ea. leg) / pg 46

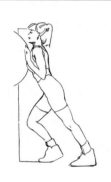

Slalom
1 Set / 1-3 Min @ 120 Bncs/Min / pg 23

Recliner
1 Set / 15 Reps / pg 23

Wall Hack Squats (Adv.)
3 Sets / 20-25 Reps ea. side / pg 28

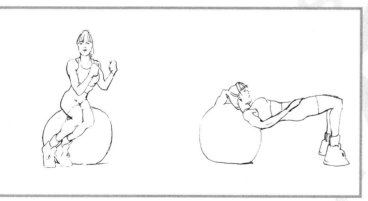

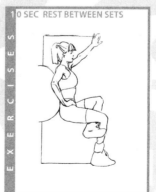

10 SEC REST BETWEEN SETS

E X E R C I S E S

Hamstring Bridges (Adv.)
20 Reps (ea. leg) / pg 29

In-'n'-Out Rolls (Adv.)
20 Reps (ea. leg) / pg 32

Glute Bridges (Beg.)
1 Set / 20 Reps (ea. leg) / pg 29

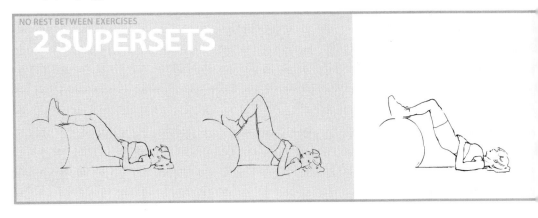

NO REST BETWEEN EXERCISES
2 SUPERSETS

Leaning Inner-Thigh Lifts
3 Sets / 20 Reps (each leg) / pg 34

Knee Squeezes (Adv.)
3 Sets / 20-25 Reps / pg 34

Side Kicks
3 Sets / 25 Reps (ea. leg) / pg 35

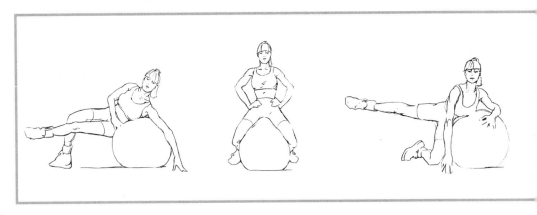

Lying Leg Thrusts
20 Reps / pg 39

Crunches
35 Reps / pg 40

Cross Crunches
30 Reps / pg 41

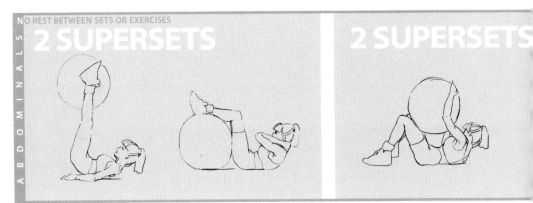

NO REST BETWEEN SETS OR EXERCISES
ABDOMINALS
2 SUPERSETS

2 SUPERSETS

Dolphins
15 Reps / pg 32

Glute Bridges (Beg.)
20 Reps / pg 29

Wall Squats (Int.)
20 Reps / pg 28

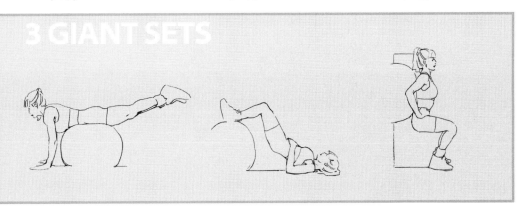

3 GIANT SETS

Leaning Calf Raises (Adv.)
3 Sets / 25-30 Reps (ea. leg) / pg 36

Supermans
15 Reps (ea. side) / pg 37

Hyperextensions
20-25 Reps / pg 37

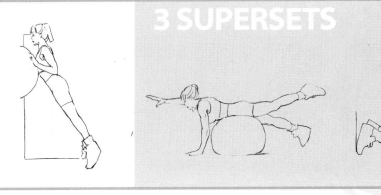

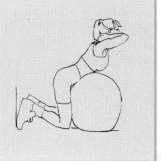

3 SUPERSETS

Crunches
35 Reps / pg 40

Springboards
2 Sets / 30 Reps / pg 42

Back Roll
1 Rep / 15-20 Sec / pg 43

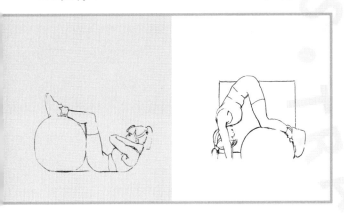

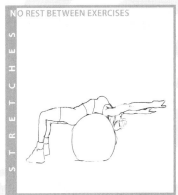

NO REST BETWEEN EXERCISES

STRETCHES

Side Stretch
1 Rep / 15-20 Sec (ea. side) / pg 44

Hamstring Stretch
1 Rep / 15-20 Sec (ea. leg) / pg 44

Swan
1 Rep / 15-20 Sec (ea. hip) / pg 45

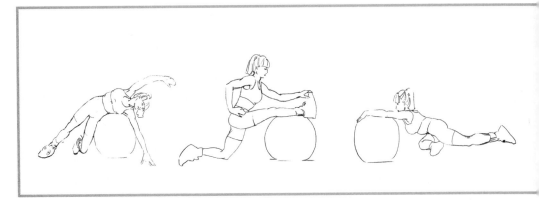

Leaning Calf Stretch
1 Rep / 15-20 Sec (ea. leg) / pg 46

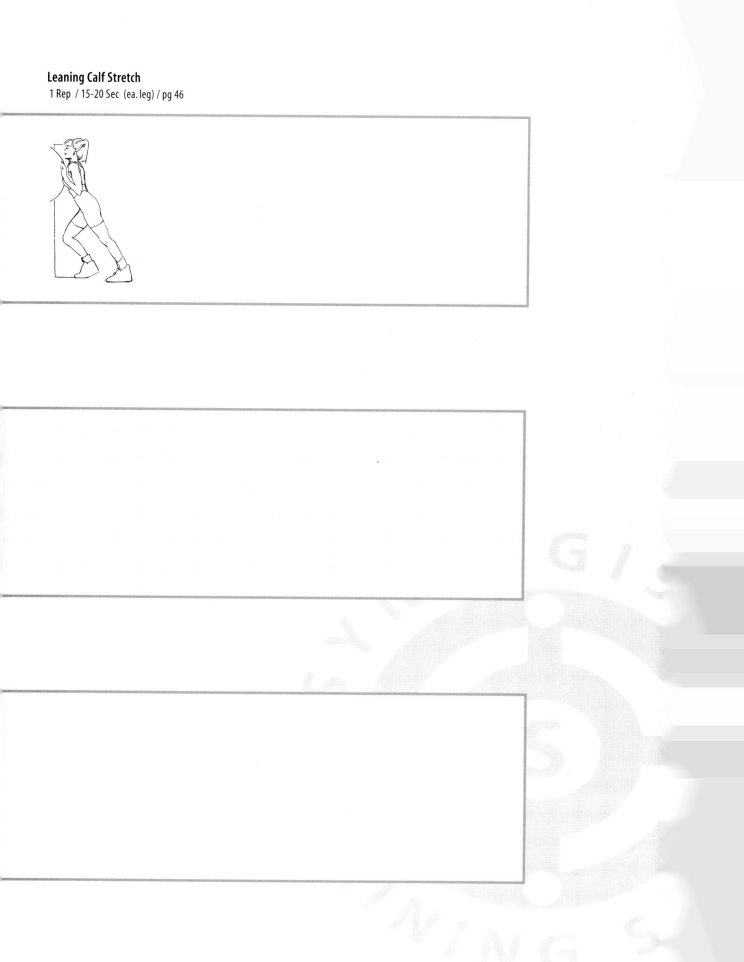

How Much, How Often

One way *HFL* programs differ from other exercise programs is that they're designed to grow with you — to get harder as you get stronger. They do this in two ways:

- by leading you through progressively harder levels
- by introducing more workouts per week

These two changes will occur at different rates, depending on your fitness level. Following the guidelines below, you may find that you move up a level before adding additional days. Or you may find you've added additional days before you move up even one level. There is no one right way to improve. What counts is sticking with the routine, marking your progress, and watching yourself get into truly terrific shape!

MOVING UP TO HIGHER LEVELS

Even if you're in pretty good shape, you should begin on *Level 1*. Use good exercise form and limit your rest to 30 seconds between sets and exercises.

When you can hit the rep goals for *Level 1* for at least four consecutive workouts, move up to *Level 2*. Likewise, when you can hit the rep goals for *Level 2* for four consecutive workouts, move up to *Level 3*, and so on. Keep in mind that there are no advantages to advancing through levels quickly! The idea is to get as much as possible out of each level before moving on.

WEEKLY SCHEDULE

An optimum workout schedule must balance work and rest. This general consideration applies regardless of your fitness level.

To that end, start by doing the *Body Ball Routine* only on Mondays and Fridays. Stick to that two-day-per-week schedule for three weeks (see schedule on the next page) even if you graduate to *Level 2*. Starting the fourth week, add a third workout on Wednesday.

Eventually, when you reach *Level 5*, you may add a fourth day. Alternate between *Levels 4* and *5* on two consecutive days followed by two days' rest, then repeat the *Level 4 / Level 5* combination on the two days after that, followed by one days' rest.

On the next two pages, you will find an idealized example of a person moving through the levels at the fastest possible rate. This is for illustrative purpose only. Following the guidelines above, advancement through the levels will naturally be much slower and will vary from person to person.

That's It!

Well, you've made it! You now have everything you need to get a highly effective work-out on your new Body Ball. If the program seems a bit complex, remember that the benefit comes from the effect of the routine *as a whole*. Your first few workouts will convince you of the power of this integrated approach.

Now it's time to inflate your Ball and get started. *Happy Training!*

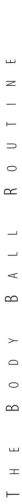

Idealized Schedule

WEEK 1						
M	T	W	Th	F	Sa	Su
L1				L1		

WEEK 2						
M	T	W	Th	F	Sa	Su
L1				L1		

WEEK 3						
M	T	W	Th	F	Sa	Su
L2				L2		

WEEK 4						
M	T	W	Th	F	Sa	Su
L2		L2		L3		

Idealized Schedule – Continued

WEEK 5						
M	T	W	Th	F	Sa	Su
L3		L3		L3		

WEEK 6						
M	T	W	Th	F	Sa	Su
L4		L4		L4		

WEEK 7						
M	T	W	Th	F	Sa	Su
L4	L5			L4	L5	

WEEK 8						
M	T	W	Th	F	Sa	Su
L4	L5			L4	L5	

Bibliography

Books

Creager, C. C., P.T., *Therapeutic Exercises Using the Swiss Ball.* Executive Physical Therapy, Boulder, CO, 1994.

Kucera, M., *Gymnastik mit dem Hupfball.* Gustav Fischer Verlag, Stuttgart, Germany, 1993.

Hypes, B., P.T., *Facilitating Development and Sensorimotor Function: Treatment With the Ball.* PDP Press, Inc., Hugo, MN, 1991.

Maurer, H., *GymnastikBall.* Ledragomma, Osoppo, Italy.

Robinson, J., *Secrets of Advanced Bodybuilders.* Health For Life, Marina del Rey, CA, 1985.

Robinson, J., *Legendary Abs.* Health For Life, Marina del Rey, CA, 1983.

Robinson, J. & Miller, R., *Transfigure I.* Health For Life, Marina del Rey, CA, 1989.

Journals / Periodicals

Brody, L., "The Axler," *Shape.* April 1993.

Carriere, P.T., CIFK, "Swiss Ball Exercises," *PT Magazine.* September 1993.

Good, N. A., P.T., "Dynamic Stabilization and Other Uses of the Therapy Balls." *The NPPTC Quarterly.* March 1993.

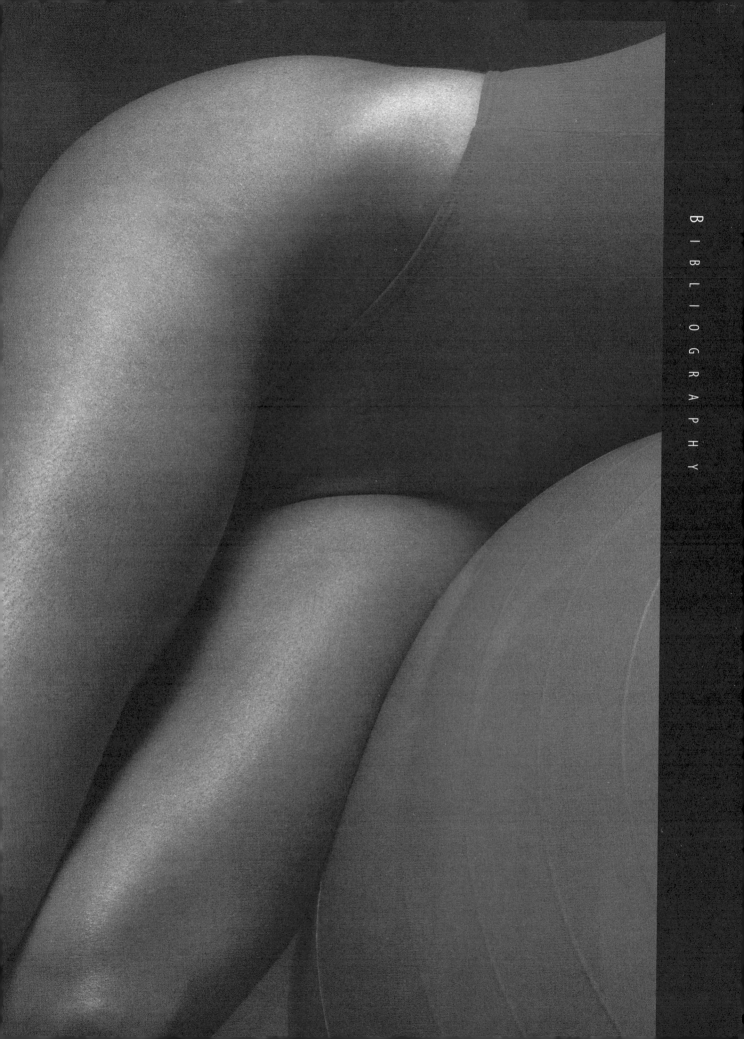

BIBLIOGRAPHY

Morgan, D., "Concepts in Functional Training and Postural Stabilization for the Low-back-Injured." *Top Acute Care Trauma Rehabilitation.* 1988; 2:8-17.

Shankman, G., A.T., C.S.C.S., "Strengthening the Lumbar Spine in Athletics," *NSCA Journal.* 1993; 15(4):15-22.

Reichley, M. L., "Roll With It: Swiss Ball Techniques," *ADVANCE for Physical Therapists.* September 6, 1993.

Videos

Klein-Vogelbach, S., *Functional Kinetics: Swiss Ball Exercises.* Springer-Verlag, New York, NY.

Morris, S.D., B.S. & Morris, M., B.S., *Get on the Ball, Resist-A-Ball.* Destin, FL. 1993.

SOME OF OUR OTHER COURSES:

THE HUMAN FUEL HANDBOOK

Health For Life's guide to peak performance nutrition, written especially for the dedicated athlete. Nutrient by nutrient, you'll discover how protein, carbohydrate, fat, minerals and vitamins function in your body...and why much of what you've heard about these substances is wrong. You'll get the real story on energy production, sports drinks, free-form amino acids, B-15, ginseng, Omega-3, steroid replacements, and much more! *Over 300 pages.*

LEGENDARY ABS

Featuring the Synergism Principle, **Legendary Abs II** guarantees rock-hard, well-defined abdominals in just 6 minutes a day! See results within two weeks, or your money back. Not isometrics or some other supposed shortcut, **Legendary Abs II** is just good science applied to bodybuilding. Over 300,000 copies sold worldwide! *A 48 p. illustrated manual.*

SYNERABS: 6 MINUTES TO A FLATTER STOMACH

Women's edition of the **Legendary Abs II** program. Guarantees a firm, well-toned midsection in just 6 minutes a day! Ten levels of routines, from beginning to advanced. *A 48 p. illustrated manual.*

TRANSFIGURE I: 9 MINUTES TO THE ULTIMATE BUTTOCKS AND THIGHS

Transfigure is a revolutionary, high-gear system of buttock and thigh conditioning, keyed to a woman's specific aesthetic goals and based on sound biomechanical principles. Forget doing hundreds of ineffective leg exercises. Get set for the fastest results you've ever experienced, with routines that allow you to take control of your body and create the lean, shapely form you want!

Transfigure includes separate routines involving body weight exercise, light resistance exercise—even competition bodybuilding work. Whether you're working for general firmness and tone, or strength and high definition, **Transfigure** is your formula for the ultimate lower body, *in just 9 minutes! 126 pp. Over 200 photographs.*

TRANSFIGURE II: FOR THE ULTIMATE UPPER BODY

Part two of our body-sculpting program for women, **Transfigure II** adds the finishing touches to the ultimate physique. It concentrates on two areas that make the biggest difference in the shape and definition of the upper body: the backs of the upper arms and the chest. It also promotes attractive, balanced development of the shoulders, back and biceps. From light-resistance exercises all the way to competition bodybuilding work...*you* select the intensity that matches your experience and goals. For all-around firmness, tone and shapely definition. *130 pp., over 100 photographs.*

SECRETS OF ADVANCED BODYBUILDERS

What **Legendary Abs** and **SynerAbs** do for abdominal conditioning, **Secrets of Advanced Bodybuilders** does for your whole workout! **Secrets** explains how to apply the Synergism Principle to training back, chest, delts, biceps, triceps, quads, and hamstrings. It unlocks the secrets of the Optimum Workout and shows you how to develop the best routines for *you*—with your particular goals, strengths, and body structure.

Get the *ultimate* program. Plus, learn... A new back exercise that will pile on the mass and increase power without putting harmful stress on your lower back • A technique for making Leg Extensions 200% more intense by targeting both inner *and outer* quads • The shift in position that cranks pull-up and pull-down exercises to three times normal intensity • A *body weight* triceps exercise that will be "a growing experience" even for someone who's been training for years • A *body weight* lat exercise that will mass up your back faster than you would have believed possible • A special shoulder set that's more effective than most entire delt routines —also— The best way to integrate your other athletic endeavors—running, cycling, stretching, mountain climbing, martial arts, etc.—into your routine to create the optimum overall program • Techniques for maximizing the effectiveness of *all* exercises you do, not just those in the course...and much, much more! *Stop working harder than you need to to get the results you want.* ***Put the* Secrets of Advanced Bodybuilders *to work for you today!*** *158 pp. Over 300 illustrations.*

MAX O$_2$: THE COMPLETE GUIDE TO SYNERGISTIC AEROBIC TRAINING

Maximize your aerobic capacity faster and with less work than ever before! **MAX O$_2$** represents an exciting new breakthrough in aerobic training. It offers a completely new perspective on the combined effect of VO$_2$ max and lactate threshold—and on the vital role this effect plays in optimum aerobic conditioning.

Learn: How the F.I.T. principle (Frequency, Intensity, and Time) can help you experience the same progress in your cardiovascular training as in other parts of your workout • How to build aerobics into any conditioning program (Bodybuilders: here's the secret to dropping bodyfat without losing muscle mass!) • Benefits and myths of cross-training • How to avoid injuries that can be caused by high-intensity aerobic work • Losing weight • Endurance events • and much, much, more! *Over 200 pages, illustrated.*

SYNERSHAPE: A SCIENTIFIC WEIGHT LOSS GUIDE

We're surrounded by weight loss myths. Crash diets. Spot reducing. Exotic herbs. Still, most plans fail, and most people who lose weight gain it back again. Is there really an honest, effective solution? **Yes!** **SynerShape** represents the next generation in awareness of how the body gains and metabolizes fat. It synthesizes the most recent findings on nutrition, exercise, and psychology into a TOTAL program, offering you the tools you need to shape the body you want.

SynerShape works. Let it work for *you! A 24 p. illustrated manual.*

THE PSYCHOLOGY OF WEIGHT LOSS

This special program-on-tape picks up where **SynerShape** leaves off. Noted psychologist Carol Landesman explores eating problems and *solutions* based on the latest research into human behavior and metabolism. Then, through a series of exercises, she helps you begin to heal the emotional conflicts behind your weight problem. **The Psychology of Weight Loss** is a unique program that brings the power of the therapy process into the privacy of your home. *A 90-minute guided introspection. On audio cassette.*

MIND GAINS

Health For Life brings you a new, effective way to master the psychological tools of peak performance. Based on the techniques which have led Eastern Bloc athletes to gold medal after gold medal, combined with the latest in Western sports psychology, **Mind Gains** is your ticket to the last frontier of physical performance.

You'll learn: How to cope with performance anxiety • How to stay motivated to succeed despite injuries, boredom, and other obstacles • How low self-esteem can sabotage your performance, and what you can do about it • How to achieve what psychologists call optimal arousal, a state in which time seems to slow and perfect technique execution occurs with ease • How to tell negative inner voices to shut up.

From proper goal setting to mental imagery rehearsals, you'll discover a wealth of new resources to increase your performance, gains, and personal satisfaction. Get the mental edge with **Mind Gains!** *150 pp. Illustrated.*

Also available: **Mind Gains** audio tape. As an accessory to the **Mind Gains** book, this guided visualization includes a relaxation phase, and a series of positive affirmations that relate specifically to athletic performance. Ideal for use before workouts, competitions, or any performance event.

THE 7-MINUTE ROTATOR CUFF SOLUTION

Almost everyone who works out experiences some kind of rotator cuff injury during a lifetime of training. Any of these injuries could spell the end of a workout career, but most can be prevented. **The 7-Minute Rotator Cuff Solution** is a quick, simple program to help prevent (or help you recover from) rotator cuff injuries. It explains in detail how the shoulder works, what can go wrong and why, and exactly what to do (and not do) to stop shoulder problems before they happen. Plus: a simple 7-minute exercise program that can eliminate shoulder pain and restore normal shoulder function in just a few weeks. *144 pp. Illustrated.*